9 STEPS THAT CAN HELP CHANGE YOUR LIFE . . .

From the authors of
THE ARTHRITIS CURE

- Consult a physician

- Take glucosamine and chondroitin sulfates to repair damaged joints.

- Improve your biomechanics to counter joint stress.

- Exercise regularly.

- Eat a healthful, joint-preserving diet.

- Maintain your ideal body weight.

- Fight depression.

- Use traditional methods to alleviate symptoms when necessary.

- Maintain a positive attitude.

THE ARTHRITIS CURE

THE MEDICAL MIRACLE THAT CAN HALT, REVERSE, AND MAY EVEN CURE OSTEOARTHRITIS

Jason Theodosakis, M.D., M.S., M.P.H.
Brenda Adderly, M.H.A. & Barry Fox, Ph.D.

St. Martin's Paperbacks

Another book by Affinity Communications Corp.

THE ARTHRITIS CURE

Copyright © 1997 by Affinity Communications Corporation.
Illustrations © 1997 by Jackie Aher.

ISBN: 0-312-96453-6

Printed in the United States of America

St. Martin's Press hardcover edition/January 1997
St. Martin's Paperbacks edition/August 1997

10 9 8 7 6 5 4 3 2 1

To my special friend Austen,
who has helped guide my life

—J.T.

Acknowledgments

◊

We'd like to thank Peter Engel, whose sore knee (and resultant sore temper) was the impetus for delving for the arthritis cure in the first place.

Also, thanks to Dr. Michael Greenberg for his persistent encouragement to share the wonderful messages contained in this book.

And we want to thank our incredible editor, Jeremy Katz, who has driven this book to success—as he will doubtless do with many others.

Important Note to Readers

◇

The material in this book is for informational purposes only. It is not intended to serve as a prescription for you, or to replace the advice of your medical doctor. Please discuss all aspects of the Arthritis Cure with your physician *before* beginning the program. If you have any medical conditions, or are taking any prescription or nonprescription medications, see your physician before beginning the program or altering or discontinuing your use of medications.

Why do we even mention the word "cure" in the same sentence with "a chronic condition"?

Our use of the word *cure* is substantiated by several references. We use the word *cure* to mean the partial or complete relief of symptoms.

Obviously, nothing in the title or content of this book is intended to suggest that the use of the recommended supplements will fully eradicate osteoarthritis. The evidence, carefully collected in this book, substantiates that the nutritional supplements recommended are frequently effective, even for long periods. Even so, we offer no guarantee that *every* individual will benefit from this program.

The laboratory analysis referred to in Chapter 4 was conducted by the University of Maryland at Baltimore. We chose this lab based on their unique familiarity with these compounds and their fine reputation as both an industry and federal research laboratory.

The university and its staff have no interest in the profit of this book; their only role is that of an independent research laboratory.

To protect their privacy, pseudonyms have been used for the individual patients mentioned in this book, and in some instances biographical details about them have been altered.

The authors of this book have no financial interest in any companies that produce, market, sell, or distribute glucosamine or chondroitin sulfate. The book was written strictly on the merits of the two supplements.

A Word from Dr. Theodosakis

I have developed and used the program described in this book with my patients and have seen impressive results. Some of these patients have been unable to get relief from or could not tolerate traditional therapies. Some remain symptom-free—even those who are no longer taking the supplements. As you read this book and decide with your doctor whether to use the supplements, you should keep in mind the following:

- Osteoarthritis is truly a variable condition; that is, two people with the same stage of cartilage damage may have different symptoms and respond differently to treatment.
- If your cartilage is worn down completely to the bone, your chances of cure are surely remote. However, the program described in this book may still offer you dramatic relief. The program is a safer and perhaps more effective treatment alternative than most standard therapies.
- Some cases of secondary osteoarthritis are reversible, and there are other medical conditions that

mimic the symptoms of osteoarthritis. By treating the underlying medical condition, the arthritic symptoms may disappear forever. Therefore, a thorough diagnosis is critical to determine the best treatment.

Contents

◇

Foreword

◇

As an orthopedic surgeon subspecializing in hip and knee joint replacement, I became frustrated with the medications available for the treatment of arthritis. One of seven surgeons at the Hendersonville Orthopedic Associates caring for people in Henderson and Transylvania Counties in North Carolina, I wanted to add another weapon to our arsenal for treating osteoarthritis. I was also interested in finding something that slowed down the progression of the disease, rather than just relieved pain.

Physicians initially believed that the nonsteroidal anti-inflammatory medications would slow the progression of osteoarthritis. Over the years, however, our experiences and more and more research showed that this is probably not the case. It seemed that none of the medications I had previously believed in truly modified the disease—they only relieved pain.

Fortunately, my research assistant gave me an article from the European literature on a new class of arthritis medications, such as glucosamine and chondroitin sulfates, called chondroprotective agents. These had been mentioned in American journals, but only as theoretical possibilities. I was delighted to find this article, which reviewed the European experience with chondroprotective agents in several thousand patients. And I was astonished to discover that there were ten double-blind glucosamine studies and eight chondroitin sulfate studies verifying the efficacy of these nutritional supplements on humans. (Glucosamine and chondroitin sulfates are not considered medications in this country.)

Excited to learn about the European success with glucosamine and chondroitin sulfate, I cautiously began to give them to my patients who were not able to tolerate nonsteroidal anti-inflammatory medications because of their side effects. These were patients who had few treatment alternatives. One patient with chronic pain in her hip, whose X rays demonstrated severe osteoarthritis, was contemplating hip replacement surgery. After taking glucosamine and chondroitin sulfate, her pain and disability had decreased significantly and she as yet has not required the surgery. Other patients suffering from severe osteoarthritis reported similar results, so I began to expand the indications of these two substances. I've been using glucosamine and chondroitin sulfate for two years now. My patients and I are gratified at the positive results.

American physicians have been criticized for their failure to use glucosamine and chondroitin sulfates. But American physicians are reluctant to use anything not proven effective in American studies, and the European data has not yet been duplicated in the United States. Why haven't there been American studies on these substances? Great question. As you'll learn from reading this book, it all boils down to money. Glucosamine and chondroitin sulfates, both natural substances, cannot be given the financial protection of a patent, so the drug companies lack financial incentives to promote them. And so the story of these two promising "osteoarthritis therapies" has not yet been told here in the United States.

I am currently conducting the first human double-blind, prospective, randomized study of these substances in the United States. We will be working with a total of 100 people suffering from mild to moderate osteoarthritis of the knee. For six months, the patients will either receive a placebo or a combination of glucosamine and chondroitin sulfates. Each participant will be evaluated for pain and disability, both before and after taking the supplements or the placebo.

Everyone with osteoarthritis, and that includes a great many people in this country and abroad, deserve to know the facts contained within this book. I congratulate Dr. Theodosakis, Dr. Fox, and Ms. Adderly for their significant contribution to the lay medical literature. It's about time!

Amal Das, M.D.

THE
ARTHRITIS
CURE

1

◇

Can Osteoarthritis Be Cured?

What is osteoarthritis?

Why is cartilage the focal point of the disease?

What are the symptoms of osteoarthritis and which joints are affected?

What causes osteoarthritis?

Who is affected by osteoarthritis?

What is the difference between osteoarthritis and rheumatoid arthritis?

How is osteoarthritis diagnosed?

What substances are being used to cure osteoarthritis?

◇

It starts with a little stiffness in your right knee. Nothing to worry about. Then you notice that the pain is getting worse, that you sometimes have trouble walking and jogging really hurts. Or perhaps there's a bit of "morning stiffness" in your hip, and it's a chore to go up and down the stairs. Something has to be done about this—you've got a life to live! You visit your doctor.

The examination is routine, hardly more than a bit of probing. As you lie on the examination table in a paper dressing gown, the doctor moves your leg up and down and from side to side. "Does it hurt when I move your leg this way?" she asks. When you nod, she says, "Hmm. I'd like to order an X ray."

The X ray shows an uneven narrowing of the joint space between the bones of your right knee. Frowning as she studies the X ray, the doctor pronounces the diagnosis: "You have osteoarthritis. You know, 'wear and tear' arthritis."

"What should I do?" you ask anxiously.

"Take aspirin or Advil for the pain," she answers reassuringly. "And don't overexercise the knee."

"But how did I get it?"

"Osteoarthritis is practically inevitable," your doctor replies. "Almost everyone your age has it. The problem is the cartilage, which protects the ends of the bones. It's wearing away, and without that cartilage to keep your bones apart, they're grinding together, causing the pain and stiffness. That's essentially all there is to osteoarthritis. We can take care of the pain, up to a point, but unfortunately, *there's nothing else we can do about it."*

The Number-One Cause of Movement Limitation

More than 50 million Americans—one in seven of us—suffer from arthritis, but almost *everyone over the age of 50 has signs of it*, if you look hard enough. Arthritis is the number-one cause of movement limitation and probably the leading cause of disability if you consider that people often become sedentary due to the associated aches and pains.

Arthritis (formerly called "degenerative joint disease") is not one disease, but a group of diseases whose common threads are that they can cause pain, inflammation, and limited movement of the joints. There are more than 100 diseases that so affect the joints, the most common of which is osteoarthritis.[1]

In a joint afflicted with osteoarthritis, the cartilage that covers and cushions the ends of the bones degenerates, allowing bones to rub together. The major symptom of osteoarthritis is pain; inflammation is usually only a problem late in the course of the disease. Up until now, doctors in the United States thought that osteoarthritis was incurable. That's why the commonly prescribed treatment is strictly palliative, designed only to relieve the pain without addressing the true causes of the disease or the condition of the joints. For mild cases, doctors prescribe painkillers such as Tylenol or nonsteroidal anti-inflammatory drugs (such as aspirin or ibuprofen, i.e., Motrin or Advil). Steroid injections (such as cortisone) and opiates are reserved for the more painful cases. Unfortunately, the painkillers and anti-inflammatories have problems. They temporarily relieve pain, but in the long run they simply cover up the symptoms while the disease progresses further. These drugs have side effects that range from the annoying to the downright dangerous—each year, thousands of people die from the adverse effects of both the anti-inflammatories and steroids. To add insult to injury, some research suggests that there is mounting evidence that nonsteroidal anti-inflammatories actually cause certain features of osteoarthritis to progress faster.[2,3,4]

So after years of masking your pain with drugs while your disease becomes progressively more severe, you may have to call in a surgeon to replace your hips or knees with artificial ones. Even with the new joint, however, you don't have as much function as you did before your arthritis developed. With surgery there's always the risk of dying or becoming permanently disabled. And surgery is painful, expensive, and not permanent—in ten years or so the replacement will begin to fail and the operation will probably have to be redone. But as the doctor said, there's nothing else to be done for osteoarthritis—or is there?

A New Approach Emerges from the Laboratories

Instead of simply dulling the pain with drugs or performing expensive and potentially dangerous surgery, many doctors in Europe and Asia (as well as a small but rapidly growing group in the United States) are actually *curing* the symptoms of osteoarthritis. They've had excellent results with approaches based on a combination of natural supplements that have been shown to *slow and eventually eliminate the disease* in many patients.

The facts about this revolutionary approach to solving a widespread problem are amazing:

• Our approach includes a combination of two nutritional supplements called *glucosamine* (glue-cose-a-mine) and *chondroitin* (con-droy-tin) *sulfates*. Both glucosamine and chondroitin sulfates are available, without a prescription, in most health food stores in America.

• Since they are substances we already consume, and produce in very small quantities in our bodies, glucosamine and chondroitin sulfates have no known significant side effects. This amazing fact stands in stark contrast to painkillers such as the nonsteroidal anti-inflammatories and cortisone injections, which can wreak havoc on the body.

• There is an extensive body of clinical research—decades' worth—proving that glucosamine and chondroitin sulfates work in both humans and animals.

• Although long used by physicians in Europe

and elsewhere, this safe and effective therapy has been overlooked by most of the American medical community. Fortunately, this is starting to change, and we are *now on the brink of a revolutionary treatment for osteoarthritis.*

The problem and its solution can be neatly summed up: Millions of Americans suffer from osteoarthritis, a painful and debilitating disease. Although most physicians consider it to be incurable, osteoarthritis can actually be stopped in its tracks or reversed by using glucosamine and chondroitin sulfates. These amazing natural substances may also be effective against other musculoskeletal conditions. This astonishing information is well known and widely accepted in many other countries across the globe. It's about time that we put it to use right here in the United States.

But can we accept medical advances that come from abroad? After all, we have a wonderful medical system. If something is that good, shouldn't we have thought of it first? Shouldn't we at least know about it?

Physicians in other countries are often ahead of us in many areas of medicine. The first heart transplant was performed in South Africa; the first "test tube" baby was born in England; France was a forerunner in the development of the AIDS drug AZT. Devices used to hold open clogged arteries, called coronary stents, are several generations more advanced in Europe than in the United States. In fact, U.S. physicians often travel to Europe to gain access to these devices for themselves or their families. We certainly have a good medical system, but it has traditionally been slow to accept new therapies or ideas. This is partially due to the Federal Drug Administration's decidedly unfriendly attitude toward the use of vitamins and other supplements for anything other than assuring that you meet your recommended daily nutritional requirements. And it's partially due to a relative lack of solid research into alternatives here in the United States. Indeed, a fair amount of the best research on alternative approaches has been conducted in Germany and other European countries. The studies are not all translated into English, so they are not widely read by physicians here in the United States. Still, it's quite surprising that a treatment used so successfully overseas for such a widespread and debilitating ailment has gone largely unnoticed in this country. Fortunately, that will soon change.

What Is Osteoarthritis?

The literal Greek translation of the word is *osteo* (of the bone), *arthro* (joint), and *itis* (inflammation). But "bone/joint inflammation" may not be the most accurate description of osteoarthritis, since joint *pain* rather than inflammation is its most important characteristic. Indeed, while inflammation is a characteristic of many forms of arthritis, it is *not* found in most cases of osteoarthritis. This may be why some physicians feel that we should call the problem *arthrosis*, which means "degenerative joint disease."

Osteoarthritis is just one of many forms of joint disease. It is, however, the most common form of arthritis, affecting the *articular cartilage*, the smooth, glistening, bluish-white substance attached to ends of the bones. (Have you ever looked at or touched the end of a chicken drumstick? That's articular cartilage.)

In addition to the articular cartilage, osteoarthritis, called OA for short, affects several other areas in and around the joints. These include:

- the subchondral bone (the ends of the bones, where the cartilage is attached)
- the capsules that surround the joints
- the muscles adjacent to the joint

Cartilage: The Focal Point of Osteoarthritis

Osteoarthritis begins in the cartilage, the rubbery, gel-like tissue found at the ends of bones. About 65 to 80 percent water, cartilage is designed to do two things: reduce the friction caused by one bone rubbing against another, and blunt the constant trauma inflicted on bones during everyday life.

Think of healthy cartilage as being something of a sponge between the hard ends of the bones. This spongy material soaks up liquid (specifically, synovial fluid) when the joint is at rest, but when the pressure is "on," the liquid is squeezed out again.

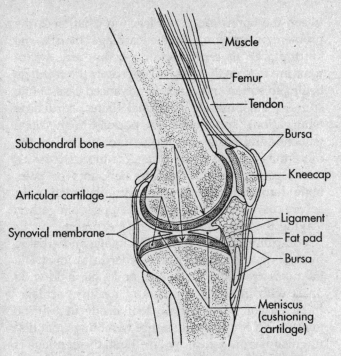

Fig. 1.1. Schematic of joint showing components.

For example, every time you take a step and the leg supports the pressure of your body weight, the cartilage in your knee joint is squeezed, forcing much of the synovial fluid out of it. But then when you pick up your foot to take another step, the fluid rushes back into the cartilage. The fluid "squishes" in and out as the cartilage responds to the constantly changing force exerted on the joint.

Over time, unfortunately, osteoarthritis can dry out the cartilage, eroding this protective buffer between the bones. As you'll learn in Chapter 2, the problem is growing in the cartilage matrix, the "birthplace" of cartilage, long before any symptoms are felt. As the disease progresses the cartilage begins to soften and crack. In advanced cases, bone spurs (osteophytes), abnormal bone hardening (eburnation), and fluid-filled pockets in the bone (subchondral cysts) can form. And, of course, the more the cartilage wears away, the more the bones rub together, creating greater amounts of pain, bone deformities, and eventually inflammation. In severe cases the cartilage may disappear altogether, leaving the bone ends completely exposed.

You can easily see cartilage damage and erosion by looking at an X ray of an osteoarthritic joint. The joint is narrowed and uneven, no longer held wide apart with the even contours of healthy cartilage. In fact, if you could actually look inside an arthritic joint, you'd immediately notice two things that distinguish it from a healthy one: First, the cartilage is breaking down, revealing an uneven, pitted surface that might even have holes in it. Second, new cartilage and new bone is being laid down by the body in an attempt to compensate for what has been lost.[5] But as you'll soon learn, this new cartilage and bone tissue can't completely replace what has been lost.

Pain, Stiffness, and Other Forms of Misery

The major symptoms of osteoarthritis are pain, stiffness, crackling, and enlargement and deformi-

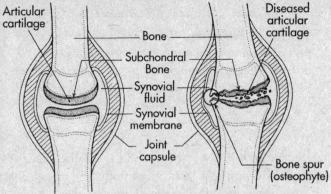

Fig. 1.2. A normal vs. osteoarthritic joint.

ties of the afflicted joint or joints, with inflammation possible in the advanced stages.

Pain. The hallmark of osteoarthritis is pain described by patients as anything from mild to moderately dull aching to deep and throbbing pain.[6] It usually begins as a minor ache that appears only after the joint has been used, and the pain often disappears with rest. But as the disease progresses, a sharp pain may strike as soon as the joint is moved or used, even a little. Eventually the joint aches even when in a resting position, unused and unpressured. In severe cases, osteoarthritic pain can disrupt sleep, making life even more miserable.

Stiffness. Osteoarthritic joints are often stiff, especially in the morning. They may also "lock up" after long periods of inactivity, such as while sitting

———————◇———————

Heberden's nodes and Bouchard's nodes are more prevalent among women between the ages of 40 and 60. They are thought to be an inherited form of osteoarthritis, since they often occur in members of the same family.

———————◇———————

in a car or a movie theater. Early in the disease process the stiffness lasts only briefly and can easily be "worked out." But as the disease worsens, a permanent loss of range of motion occurs that does not change, even with warm-up exercises and continual motion.

Joint Crackling. Also known as *crepitus*, this crackling and crunching feeling emanating from the affected joint(s) (most often a knee and less commonly a hip) occurs in advanced stages of osteoarthritis. It may be caused by the joints rubbing together during regular use, or when the joint is passively manipulated during a medical examination. Most often striking the knees, the "creaking" sound can sometimes be heard all the way across a room! As frightening as it sounds, however, it's usually painless or, at most, accompanied by only a dull sensation.[7]

Deformity and Joint Enlargement/Inflammation. As the cartilage degenerates, as the bones become damaged and the body's regulatory mechanisms fail, the afflicted joint may become deformed. Bone spurs may twist the joint's contours, making it difficult to move the bones. Heberden's nodes can disfigure the joints of the fingers closest to the fingertips, while Bouchard's nodes can cause enlargement of the middle joints of the fingers.[8] There may also be bone cysts, gross bony overgrowth, bowed legs, and knock knees. Fluid retention can also be a problem. In some cases, a doctor may have to take out as much as 100 milliliters of fluid (about four ounces) from a single osteoarthritic joint.

Although osteoarthritis can strike any joint, its "favorite" targets are the fingers, weight-bearing joints such as the knees and hips, the neck, lower back, and some joints in the feet. It can appear in one or more joints anywhere in the body, in no particular order, but usually does not strike symmetrically (that is, not in *both* hips or *both* knees, at least not at first).

Primary Versus Secondary Osteoarthritis

Osteoarthritis appears in two distinct forms—*primary* and *secondary. Primary osteoarthritis*, the more common form, is a slow and progressive condition that usually strikes after the age of 45, affecting mostly the weight-bearing joints of the knees and hips, as well as the lower back, neck, and fingers. Primary osteoarthritis develops in two ways: when excessive loads are placed on normal joint tissues

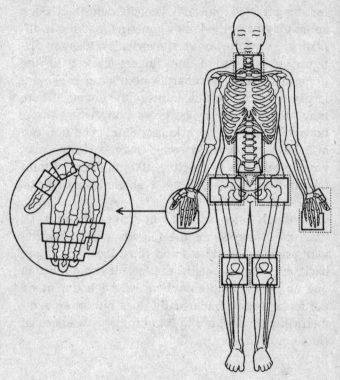

Fig. 1.3. Joints commonly affected by osteoarthritis.

(cartilage and subchondral bone), or when a reasonable load is applied on inferior joint tissues. The exact cause of primary osteoarthritis has not yet been determined, although family history and obesity are known risk factors.

The famous Framingham Heart Study, which began more than 36 years ago, was primarily designed to identify the causes of heart disease. But

———————◇———————

Under everyday, normal circumstances, cartilage is subjected to heavy impact loading, which it handles very well.

———————◇———————

it also looked into the genesis of osteoarthritis, finding a conclusive link between this disease and obesity. The acclaimed study showed that obese people are more likely to develop osteoarthritis than are their slim counterparts. And no wonder! The knees and hips, which are the primary weight-bearing joints of the body, handle loads up to 2.5 to 10 times a person's body weight. This means that if you weigh 200 pounds, some of your joints may be handling as much as a ton of pressure as you walk, run, or otherwise use them. Clearly, the load on your joints can become incredibly difficult to bear as your body weight increases. Researchers have found that middle-aged women can greatly reduce the risk of developing osteoarthritis simply by losing weight.[9, 10]

Heredity also appears to play a role in the development of primary osteoarthritis. As many as six million osteoarthritis sufferers can thank defective DNA for their aches and pains. A study of nineteen members of a single family, spanning three generations, helped researchers identify the mutation of a gene on the twelfth chromosome that they think may be associated with osteoarthritis.[11]

Secondary osteoarthritis is quite different than the primary form. It often appears before the age of 40

————————◇————————

Not all high-stress activities damage the joints.
For example, the graceful divers of Acapulco who
daily plunge from heights of more than 100 feet
do not suffer from osteoarthritis of the spine.
Scientists can offer no explanation for the divers'
apparent immunity.

————————◇————————

and has clearly defined causes: trauma or injury, joint laxity (a loose or "trick" knee, for example), joint infection, metabolic imbalances (like gout or calcium deposits, or due to chronic use of certain medications), or even just joint surgery.

Trauma appears to be the main culprit in secondary osteoarthritis, especially in younger people. The trauma can be *acute* (such as a sudden, serious injury) or *chronic* (recurring over time). Chronic trauma causes cumulative damage to the joint, one little "ouch" after another. The individual "ouches" may not be particularly severe, but added together over long periods of time, they can cause the joint tissues to fail. You'll often see chronic trauma in a joint that's unstable or "loose" because a supporting ligament was torn sometime in the past.

Repetitive impact loading is another form of chronic trauma. Repetitive impact loading involves repeated motions that traumatize the joint. A baseball pitcher throwing a ball hundreds of thousands of times, a pneumatic drill operator absorbing the vibrations of his drill in his shoulders for years, and a ballerina going from a flat foot to standing on her toes can all suffer from repetitive impact loading. Given time, these repeated motions can damage the cartilage and subchondral bone and cause secondary osteoarthritis. Repetitive impact loading is a major cause of secondary osteoarthritis, especially in joints already suffering from abnormal alignment or that are used in ways that they aren't meant to be.

Your osteoarthritis may also be caused by poor bone alignment, joints that are not formed "quite right," or by something as simple as the way you walk. Using advanced computer technology and high-speed video cameras, doctors can analyze what's happening inside your joints. They can find out how well your joints function under pressure, whether there are biological abnormalities, if your gait or stride length is contributing to your osteoarthritis, and how walking or running on different surfaces affects your joints. If what's "bugging" your joints is simply that they're being stressed in an abnormal way, your doctor and physical therapist can devise special ways of "unloading" them— or removing excessive pressure. Techniques for taking a load off your joints include:[12]

- Brief periods of rest.
- Using a cane in the hand on the side opposite the affected lower extremity joint.
- Losing weight, if necessary.
- Using soft neck collars, shoulder slings, splints on

the wrists or fingers, and back corsets for brief periods of acute pain.

Who Is Affected by Osteoarthritis?

Osteoarthritis afflicts countless millions of people worldwide, including more than 50 million Americans.[13] It strikes all animals with bony skeletons, including birds, amphibians, and reptiles—even underwater mammals such as whales and porpoises.[14] And it seems as if osteoarthritis has plagued just about anything with bones since the beginning of time. The famous Roman baths were originally used to ease the pain of arthritic joints. Archaeologists have found evidence of osteoarthritis in Egyptian mummies, and paleontologists discovered it in the skeletons of early man dating back half a million years. In fact, the dinosaurs had it 200 million years ago.

Between 33 and 66 percent of any given group of people are afflicted with osteoarthritis.[15] The statistics vary, but it's fair to say that about 2 percent of those under the age of 45, 30 percent of those between 45 and 64, and 63 to 85 percent of those over the age of 65 suffer from osteoarthritis.[16] The true numbers may actually be higher, for many people with osteoarthritis have not yet developed symptoms. Among osteoarthritis victims under age 45, secondary osteoarthritis is more common, while primary osteoarthritis is rare.

Men are more likely to suffer from osteoarthritis

---◇---

Osteoarthritis patterns vary according to ethnic background. For example, osteoarthritis of the hips is rarely seen in Japan and Saudi Arabia but is quite common in the United States.

---◇---

than are women up to the age of 45, perhaps because males tend to engage in more strenuous physical activities. From age 45 to 55, however, men and women begin to have an equal chance of suffering, while women are more likely victims after the age of 55. Not only is osteoarthritis more frequent in women age 55 or older, it is also more severe. Millions of women of all ages have osteoarthritis and are affected twice as often as men.

Osteoarthritis Is Not Rheumatoid Arthritis

Osteoarthritis and rheumatoid arthritis are often confused because their names are similar and they both afflict the joints. But they are very different diseases. Rheumatoid arthritis is an immune-system disorder that can lead to weakness, fatigue, fever, anemia, and other problems, including inflamed joints. (An immune-system disorder is one in which the body attacks its own tissues, as if they were foreign invaders.) Rheumatoid arthritis tends to strike symmetrically, which means that it hits both sides of the body at once (both wrists, both hands, and so on). Some two and a half million people in the United States have rheumatoid arthritis.[17] Here are some of the major distinctions between osteoarthritis and the far less common rheumatoid arthritis:

Osteoarthritis	Rheumatoid Arthritis
Usually begins after age 40.	Initially strikes between the ages of 25 and 50.
Develops gradually over several years.	Often comes and goes without warning.
Usually begins in joints on one side of the body.	Usually attacks joints on both sides of the body simultaneously (e.g., both hands).
Redness, warmth, and swelling (inflammation) of joints is unusual.	Redness, warmth, and swelling (inflammation) of joints is almost universal.
Primarily affects joints of the knees, hands, hips, feet, and spine. Only occasionally attacks the knuckles, wrists, elbows, or shoulders.	Affects many or most joints, including the knuckles, wrists, elbows, and shoulders.
Doesn't cause an overall feeling of sickness.	Often causes an overall feeling of sickness and fatigue, as well as weight loss and fever.[18]

Diagnosing the Joint Malady

Before making a diagnosis of osteoarthritis, a good doctor will carefully note your complaints, review

———————◇———————

Fine hand movements such as pinching are not usually affected by osteoarthritis.

———————◇———————

your medical history, and examine you from head to toe. During the examination he or she will look for several distinct signs, such as limited range of motion in the joints, tenderness to touch (palpation), pain upon bending and flexing your joint (passive motion), and joint crackling and grinding (crepitus).

Limited Range of Motion in the Joints. At first the inability to move a joint as well as before may be subtle and hard to measure, but with time the limitation of movement becomes obvious. If the osteoarthritis is in the hand, for example, you may have difficulty opening a jar or grasping a ball. If it's in the knee, bending or extending the joint can become very uncomfortable. If your spine is affected, you may have trouble twisting or bending. And if the problem is severe enough, the weight-bearing joints of the hips and knees may not be well enough for you to do simple activities.

Tenderness to Touch. The joint may not feel tender at all in the early stages of the disease, but it can swell as the body produces more fluid in the joint. The excess fluid puts pressure on the tissues surrounding the joint, which causes pain and tenderness to touch.

———————◇———————

Osteophytes, which can be seen on an X ray, are considered to be a sign that the bone is trying to repair itself in order to support the load on an affected joint.

———————◇———————

Pain with Passive Motion. We don't normally know if we have pain upon passive motion because our movement is almost always active. It's usually only when a doctor moves our arms and legs about that we experience passive movement. Many times, however, we'll feel pain, and a crunching or creaking of the bones when the doctor manually bends and flexes our afflicted joints.

In addition to checking for these physical signs of osteoarthritis, the doctor will request a simple X ray to confirm the diagnosis. Osteoarthritis shows up on an X ray first by changes in the bone just beneath the cartilage. Narrowing of the joint spaces is often seen as well. In advanced cases, bones spurs, abnormal denseness, and pockets of fluid in the bone may also be apparent. More sophisticated imaging techniques, such as arthroscopy, CT (computerized tomography) scans, and MRI (magnetic resonance imaging), may also be used to help assess the extent of cartilage damage.[19]

What Does Not Cause Osteoarthritis?

Despite plenty of evidence to the contrary, three common misconceptions about osteoarthritis persist: that it is a normal part of the aging process, that it is a "wear and tear" disease, and that it cannot be halted or reversed. Nothing could be further from the truth!

• *Osteoarthritis is* not *inevitable.* We used to believe that the joint deterioration found with aging was the same kind of deterioration seen in those with osteoarthritis. Now we know that there are striking differences between joints and cartilage that are affected by osteoarthritis and those that have simply aged normally.[20, 21] These differences are described below:

Aged Joints	Osteoarthritic Joints
Deterioration occurs on *non-*weight-bearing cartilage surfaces.	Deterioration occurs on weight-bearing cartilage surfaces.
Minimal physical and chemical changes in the cartilage matrix.	Significant physical, chemical, and degradative changes in the cartilage matrix.
No increase in tissue volume.	Increase in tissue volume.
No change in the liquid content of the cartilage.	Early and dramatic increase in the liquid content of cartilage. (This may be the first physical change.)
Pigment in cartilage.	No pigment in cartilage.
No eburnation (excess bone denseness or overgrowth).	Eburnation.
No obvious bone changes.	Bone changes, including new bone formation (osteophytes).

While it is true that osteoarthritis occurs more frequently and severely in older persons, this is due to prolonged exposure to the everyday traumas and repetitive motions that occur throughout a lifetime and a decrease in the ability for minor self-repair. While osteoarthritis may occur more often and with more severity as we age, it is not *caused* by the aging process.

• *Primary osteoarthritis is* not *caused by wear and tear on the body, due to strenuous activity or exercise.* Recent scientific studies have conclusively proven that regular exercise does not predispose us to osteoarthritis. In fact, the opposite is true: vigorous exercise actually *increases* the functional status in those with osteoarthritis.[22] Secondary arthritis due to injuries or repetitive impact loading may be caused by use and abuse of a joint, but normal amounts of exercise actually help to *prevent* primary arthritis, and can play a major role in treating the disease.

• *We* can *relieve the pain and disability of osteoarthritis.* Most doctors in the United States shrug their shoulders and accept the "inevitable" when treating patients with osteoarthritis, prescribing nothing more than painkillers. But advances in the understanding of cartilage and years of experience with numerous patients have shown that it is definitely possible to slow, halt, or prevent the degeneration of cartilage that is characteristic of osteoarthritis.[23] Specifically, there is strong evidence suggesting that restoring the normal balance to the cartilage matrix can have a positive impact on the course and outcome of the disease.[24]

The traditionally minded American medical establishment has turned a deaf ear to the exciting studies pouring forth from research centers and hospitals all over Europe and Asia. But this growing body of evidence is beginning to force doctors to reevaluate their thinking, to open their minds to the promise of glucosamine and chondroitin sulfates. They are slowly beginning to realize that osteoarthritis is *not* inevitable, and that it may even be cured.

There Is Hope

Osteoarthritis is a very common affliction that most doctors in the United States think is both inevitable and incurable. Fortunately, they are wrong! The Arthritis Cure has helped to relieve the pain of osteoarthritis for many people around the world, allowing them to once again enjoy normal and productive lives.

2

When Joints Go Bad

How does a joint work?

What is cartilage made of?

What happens when cartilage degenerates?

Can damaged cartilage be healed without surgery or exotic and possibly dangerous medicines?

Shoulders, knees, elbows, hips, fingers, and more—the human body has 143 different joints, parts of which act as the hinges, levers, and shock absorbers that allow us to stand, walk, run, kneel, jump, dance, climb, sit, grasp, push, pull, shake hands, scratch our heads, eat, and otherwise perform the thousands of motions that get us through the day. Whether it's a large knee joint or a little toe joint, each is a complex unit that makes movement possible. These mechanical marvels hold bones close enough together to allow coordinated movement, while ensuring that they slide gently over each other, never sticking or grinding.

Three Types of Joints

All of the joints in the human body fall into one of three categories: fixed, slightly moveable, or highly mobile. The differences in our joints allow us to achieve the perfect balance between stability and movement.

Fixed joints join together bones that have very little, if any, movement against each other, such as the suture joints that connect the bony plates that form the skull. Arthritis is not a problem in these stationary joints, which are called synarthrodial (sin-arth-ro-dial) joints.

Slightly moveable joints bring together bones that can move a little bit with respect to each other, such as the sacroiliac joints, which connect the lowest part of the spine with the pelvis (thus connecting the upper and lower body). Called amphiarthroidal (am-fee-arth-roid-al) joints, they only occasionally succumb to osteoarthritis.

It's the highly mobile joints that are the chief targets of osteoarthritis. Also called diarthroidal (die-arth-roid-al) or synovial (sin-o-vee-ol) joints, they come in many different forms. The elbows, for example, are *hinge joints* that allow the lower arms to swing up to meet the upper arms, much like a door swings open and closed. The *ball-and-socket* joints that connect the upper leg bones to the pelvis allow for a much wider range of motion than the hinge joints. You can move your legs forward and backward, to the left and to the right, or even around in a semicircular manner. Then there are *saddle joints* that bring together the bones at the base of the thumbs, *gliding joints* in the hand, carpal bones, and more.

Highly mobile joints come in many different sizes and shapes, though they all have similar purposes and structures. They are designed to hold bones very close together while allowing them to move smoothly against each other. Their structure, although complex, is much the same whether it be a hinge, ball-and-socket, saddle, or other type of highly mobile joint. These joints have:

- *The joint capsule*—a tough membrane or "sack" that encloses the joint and connects one bone to another, holding them firmly in place;
- *Synovium*—the inner lining of the joint capsule, which secretes *synovial fluid* to lubricate as well as to nourish the cartilage;
- *Cartilage*—which caps the ends of the bones and absorbs shock, while providing a slick surface so that the bone ends can easily glide across each other during movement;
- *Ligaments*—which attach bones to bones, and help provide stability;
- *Tendons*—which attach muscles to bones, allow

for movement, and act as secondary joint stabilizers;
- *Muscles*—which contract to provide the force for movement and are critical for much of the shock absorption around a joint; and
- *Bursae*—small, fluid-filled sacs positioned at strategic points to cushion ligaments and tendons, protecting them against friction and wear and tear.

A Closer Look at Articular Cartilage

We're primarily concerned with the cartilage in the joints. There are many types of cartilage performing many different functions in the body, but the cartilage found in the joint is *articular* cartilage. Since this is the "magic" substance that must be present and healthy for smooth, pain-free movement in the joints, it's worth taking the time to examine it in greater detail.

To get an idea of what cartilage does, imagine rubbing together two perfectly flat, smooth, slightly wet ice cubes. They glide across each other quickly and easily, never catching or slowing. Now imagine a surface that's five to eight times *more* slippery than ice. That's your cartilage, the material that makes it possible for the ends of your bones to slide smoothly and easily across each other. In fact, no man-made substance can compare to the low-friction and shock-absorbing properties of healthy cartilage.

—————◇—————

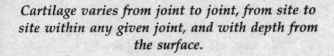

Cartilage varies from joint to joint, from site to site within any given joint, and with depth from the surface.

—————◇—————

Like much of the body, cartilage is a watery substance—in fact, it's 65 to 80 percent water.[1] The rest of it is made up of *collagen* and *proteoglycans*, the substances that give cartilage its amazing properties of resilience and shock absorption. Together, water, collagen, and proteoglycans form the *cartilage matrix*, the "birthplace" of cartilage.

Collagen, a protein known for its versatility, is found in many different parts of the body, taking different forms to fulfill various functions. Collagen is altered into strong ropes to make tendons, thin sheets to form skin, clear membranes to make corneas, and strong, weight-bearing structures that we call bones. Collagen is a vital part of cartilage, providing it with elasticity and the ability to absorb shock. It also creates a framework to hold the proteoglycans in place.[2] In a sense, collagen is the "glue" that holds the cartilage matrix together.

Proteoglycans are huge molecules made up of protein and sugars. Looking a little like round bottle brushes, proteoglycans are woven around and through the collagen fibers, forming a dense netting inside the cartilage. The proteoglycans make cartilage resilient so that it can stretch then bounce back when we move.[3] The amazing proteoglycans also trap water. Imagine that you're holding a sponge

---

◇

"Healthy proteoglycans look like fresh Christmas trees; in osteoarthritis they are as scraggly as cast-off trees in February."
—Harvard Health Letter, 1992

◇

---

under water. When you squeeze that sponge water squirts out, only to rush back in as soon as you relax your grip. Thanks to the thirsty and resilient proteoglycans, your cartilage acts like that sponge, rapidly absorbing water when the pressure is off the joint, then squeezing it out again when the pressure is on. This allows cartilage to respond to our movements and absorb shock without cracking under the strain, the way a solid material would.

In addition to the collagen and proteoglycans, there are also special cells called *chondrocytes* sprinkled throughout the cartilage matrix. Chondrocytes are miniature factories that produce new collagen and proteoglycan molecules, always making sure that there are enough of these vital substances.[4] But since everything eventually ages and weakens, the chondrocytes also release enzymes to "chew up" and dispose of the aging collagen and proteoglycan molecules that have passed their prime.

When Physical Stress Damages Cartilage

These four elements of healthy cartilage—collagen, proteoglycans, chondrocytes, and water—work together to ensure smooth, pain-free movement. Unfortunately, several things can disrupt the careful teamwork, causing disease and painful distress. We don't know exactly what causes *primary osteoarthritis*, but we do know that *secondary osteoarthritis* is often caused by trauma.[5] The trauma may be sudden and severe, such as a blow to the hip while playing football. Or perhaps the trauma is slow and gradual, the built-up effects of hundreds or thousands of tiny injuries. Obesity can also damage joints by forcing them to bear too much weight. Or joints may become damaged simply because a person has inherited a body that "wears" in an unfortunate manner. Whatever the reason, when the trauma occurs, the once-healthy cartilage may begin to break down.

The surface of damaged cartilage may become ragged and pockmarked, eventually wearing through completely, leaving holes that make it look like a motheaten sweater. Without healthy and whole cartilage to cushion them, the bones may begin to rub against each other, causing severe pain. Or small fractures may develop in the cartilage. The body usually responds to this by producing more cartilage to "plug the cracks," but the replacement cartilage is often inferior in quality, unable to cushion the bone ends against the forces of impact. As a result, the ends of those bones change, losing some of their ability to "bend" under stress and act as shock absorbers. The body may overproduce bone material for the bone ends in an attempt to correct the problem, but that can lead to bumpy surfaces in the joint.

Whether it's the cartilage or the bone that's damaged, the result is trouble. Damaged, uneven cartilage is like a scraggly old carpet, and an overgrown bone is like a floor littered with sharp rocks. In either case, the joint no longer has smooth contours, so fluid, pain-free movement is impossible.

As the joint degenerates, the joint lining (synovium) often becomes inflamed. The synovium has many nerve endings and pain receptors, so inflammation invariably sends pain messages rocketing off to the brain. The synovium tries to solve the problem by producing more and more synovial fluid, the slick watery substance that lubricates and nourishes the cartilage. This sounds like a good idea, but the resulting fluid ends up flooding the joint space, causing swelling and perhaps even more pain. The synovium itself may also swell up and exude a puslike material.

That's what's happening inside the ailing joint. But all you are aware of is that your knee really hurts, it's swollen, it's hard to bend, and you don't want to put weight on it. And all this began with some type of triggering event.

Theories for the Primary Form of Osteoarthritis

We know that physical stress is one cause of *secondary osteoarthritis*, but researchers have yet to determine the exact cause of *primary osteoarthritis*. Several theories have been developed to explain the genesis of this painful and puzzling problem.

1. *There may be changes in the cartilage matrix.* The chondrocytes are responsible for maintaining the normal mix of collagen, proteoglycans, and water that make up the cartilage matrix. For unknown reasons, the "recipe" gets scrambled, the proportions altered. The body tries to correct the problem by making more chondrocytes, which in turn churn out greater amounts of collagen and proteoglycans. Unfortunately, excess fluid also builds up, "washing away" these newly synthesized molecules—and possibly older ones, as well—leaving fewer than ever.[6]

2. *An unchecked enzyme in the cartilage may be out of control.* Chondrocytes produce collagen and proteoglycans, so the body may try to correct cartilage problems by manufacturing more chondrocytes. But the chondrocytes don't limit themselves to making cartilage-building materials— they also make enzymes that break down old collagen and proteoglycans. Extra chondrocytes means more "cartilage-building" substances *and* more "cartilage-busting" enzymes. The net result may be the opposite of what was intended, with more cartilage being destroyed than created. When a joint is flooded with these cartilage-chewing enzymes, the collagen fibers in the cartilage become smaller, and the dense netting that they provide relaxes. The proteoglycans,

which are normally held in place by the collagen, begin to drift off and disappear. Without
enough proteoglycans around to attract and
hold water, the cartilage dries out and becomes
more susceptible to cracking, fissuring, and
wearing through completely.

These cartilage-busting enzymes that the chondrocytes produce are normally kept in check by
an equal number of cartilage-promoting enzymes. If the balance is off, or if too many of the
cartilage-destroying enzymes are produced, the
results can be disastrous.[7]

3. *Trauma to the subchondral bone can trigger the problem.* The portion of the bone located directly under the cartilage may be damaged by an injury
or by repeated stress to the joint. This could lead
to a cycle of bony overgrowth and joint damage.

4. *Bone disease may be the culprit.* A problem with
the blood supply could weaken the bone, leading to small fractures and *osteonecrosis*, which
means "bone death." Alcoholism, infection, and
acute trauma are among the possible culprits in
this scenario.[8]

5. *Abnormal liver function may be a cause.* The liver
(source of many hormones, growth factors, and
substances that aid cartilage and bone formation) may not function properly, resulting in
bony overgrowth and cartilage destruction.

Whatever the cause may be, all OA sufferers
seem to want to know the same things: Can the
damage be repaired? Is there a way to make the

cartilage surface slick and slippery again? Is it possible to repair and restore cartilage that was damaged long ago? Would fixing the cartilage cure the pain, inflammation, and bony overgrowth? And would that cure the arthritis?

We believe that the answer to all of these questions is a resounding yes! This is the basis of the "chondroprotective" theory of treating arthritis, an approach based on protecting cartilage cells. It *is* possible to stop the destruction of cartilage in osteoarthritis, to repair some of the lost cartilage, and to improve joint function. We *can* restore health and balance to the cartilage matrix without waiting for complex new surgeries or new substances to be perfected. Along with the rest of our program, we *can* often reduce or eliminate the pain and disability of osteoarthritis with two simple nutritional supplements: glucosamine and chondroitin sulfates.

3

◊

New Hope for Beating Osteoarthritis

What is glucosamine? How does it work?

*What are chondroitin sulfates?
How do they work?*

*Why are glucosamine and chondroitin sulfates
used together?*

*How do glucosamine and chondroitin fare in
scientific studies?*

*Are there other substances that work with
glucosamine and chondroitin?*

*Why has it taken so long for glucosamine and
chondroitin to be used in the United States?*

*Do I need a prescription to buy glucosamine and
chondroitin sulfates? And where can they be
purchased?*

◊

Slim, well-toned 42-year-old Brett Jacobs was an exuberant amateur athlete. Although he worked hard at his job as vice president of advertising at a large toy firm, he still managed to jog several days a week, play basketball with the guys on Thursday nights, and pitch for the company softball team on the weekends.

And then one day his right knee began to hurt. It was a dull, aching pain on the inside of his knee that came and went for no apparent reason. At first it only struck while he was jogging or running up and down the basketball court, but soon he began to feel it while standing still, sitting at his desk, and finally even when he was sleeping. There was no pattern to the pain, except that it was steadily growing worse.

Fortunately, he had excellent medical insurance and was seen by the best orthopedists, neurologists, rheumatologists, internists, chiropractors, acupuncturists, and other specialists. But the exhaustive (although noninvasive) testing found absolutely nothing wrong with his knees—or with any other part of his body, for that matter. He took various pain medications, had physical therapy, and even got a steroid injection. Frustrated, he finally had arthroscopic surgery and was found to have some cartilage degeneration on the end of his thigh bone (femur). The surgeon felt that there was nothing that could be done surgically, especially since Brett's cartilage had not yet completely worn through. He essentially told Brett to "grin and bear it." But the pain grew continually worse, and within a year Brett had given up jogging, basketball, and baseball. He certainly wasn't grinning anymore.

Less than two years after the first mild pain appeared, Brett was forced to spend most of his day sitting in a chair, only standing and moving about when absolutely necessary. Luckily, his job allowed him to sit at a desk most of the day. But he missed his active life. When his friends would ask him if he'd ever be able to join them in sports again, he would sigh heavily and say: "No, I'm hanging up my running shoes. My old life as an active person is over, and now I'm the gold-medal champion sitter-downer. But the good news is that with all the aspirin I'm taking for my knee, there's no chance I'll ever have another headache."

Depressed, Brett had given up all hope of ever being able to walk without pain. Then he heard about glucosamine and chondroitin on a radio show about health and nutrition. They were only mentioned briefly, but Brett decided to give them a try. Two weeks after he started taking glucosamine and chondroitin sulfates, he said, "I stopped taking the aspirin, just to see what would happen. I was surprised to see that my knee didn't hurt much anymore. So I started standing up and walking around a little, just a little. I kept taking the glucosamine and chondroitin. A couple weeks after that I started pushing it, walking all the way around the block, just to see what would happen.

It was great, no pain! I added a little more activity every week. One week I increased my walking to ten minutes a day, the next week to fifteen, the next to twenty. Then I added in riding the bicycle at the club for five minutes, the next week for ten minutes, and so on. Little by little I did more and more until I was actually jogging again. Only a mile at first, but I was actually doing it! Then I started adding in a little baseball, then a little basketball, then a little more, and a little more. Now I'm doing just about everything I used to do."

Six months after he started taking glucosamine and chondroitin sulfates, Brett was once again lacing on his jogging shoes, playing weekend softball, and "shooting hoops" with his friends. "I'm 90 percent back," he now says with a grin, "hoping to be 100 percent soon!"

Patients aren't the only ones raving about these two arthritis-busting nutritional supplements. Doctors in Europe and Asia have been successfully using glucosamine and chondroitin sulfates for years to treat osteoarthritis. Fortunately, doctors across the United States are learning about these supplements, little by little, and prescribing them for their patients with excellent results.

Just Imagine

Healthy cartilage needs three things: water for lubrication and nourishment, proteoglycans to attract

and hold the water, and collagen to keep the proteoglycans in place.

Imagine a dense netting made up of countless
ropes woven together, some going up and down,
others running from side to side to form a mesh.
Healthy cartilage has a similar structure. Its
"threads" are tough, ropy collagen, laid down at
right angles to each other in a crisscross pattern,
four layers thick.

Proteoglycans anchor themselves securely in
place in the spaces in the collagen "netting" by
wrapping themselves over, under, around, and
through the collagen threads. The proteoglycans
are absolutely essential for healthy cartilage, for
they attract and hold many times their weight in
water, which both lubricates and nourishes the cartilage. But if the cartilage is damaged, or if the cartilage-chewing enzymes go wild, the "netting"
becomes weak. As the "netting" loses its shape and
"stretches out," proteoglycans lose their grip and
float away. Without these water-attracting molecules in place, the cartilage loses its ability to absorb shock, which makes it more susceptible to
cracking, fissuring, and possibly even wearing
through completely.

Building the "Water Holders"

How does glucosamine figure into healthy cartilage? Glucosamine is a major building block of the

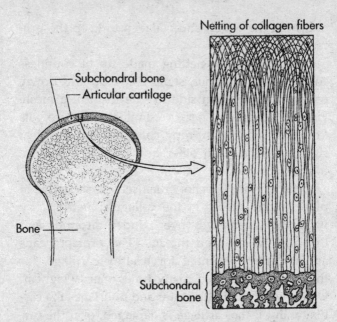

Fig. 3.1. Composition and structure of cartilage.

water-loving proteoglycans. Specifically, glucosamine is needed to make the *glycosaminoglycans* (*GAGs*), proteins that bind water in the cartilage matrix. Besides providing raw material for the synthesis of proteoglycans and GAGs, glucosamine's mere presence acts as a stimulant to the cells that produce these products, the *chondrocytes*.[1] In fact, glucosamine has been found to be the key factor in determining how many proteoglycans are produced by the chondrocytes. If there is a lot of glucosamine present, then a lot of proteoglycans will be produced, and a lot of water will be held in its

———————◇———————

Glucosamine is made up of glucose, the sugar that the body burns for fuel, and an amino acid called glutamine. It is an important part of the mucopolysaccharides, which provide structure to the bone, cartilage, skin, nails, hair, and other body tissues.

———————◇———————

proper place. But if only a little glucosamine is available, fewer proteoglycans will be made, and less of the precious water will be attracted to the area. Glucosamine has also been shown to spur the chondrocytes to produce more collagen and proteoglycans, and it also normalizes cartilage metabolism, which helps to keep the cartilage from breaking down.[2]

Because glucosamine "jump-starts" the production of these key elements of the cartilage matrix, and then protects them, *it can actually help the body to repair damaged or eroded cartilage.* In other words, glucosamine strengthens your body's natural repair mechanisms.

Several studies have shown that besides stimulating the production of cartilage, glucosamine helps to reduce pain and improve joint function in those with osteoarthritis.[3,4] And it doesn't seem to matter if the glucosamine is manufactured by the body or comes from a supplement. Supplemental glucosamine acts just like the glucosamine that we eat in very small quantities in our food and the

———————◇———————

*Glucosamine continues to work even after the
treatment stops.*

———————◇———————

glucosamine found naturally in our cartilage.
Where it comes from doesn't seem to matter. It just
needs to be *present*.

In the United States, glucosamine supplements
are available as nonprescription items in four
forms—hydrochloride, hydroiodide, n-acetyl, and
sulfate. Regulated and sold as a drug in Europe,
glucosamine sulfate is the form that is used in most
research. Although the sulfate form is used most
often, other forms may work just as well. Those
with thyroid conditions should avoid the hydroiodide form.

The Proof Is in the Lack of Pain

Theoretically, glucosamine should be a powerful
osteoarthritis remedy. But theory and actual practice do not always agree, which is why theories are
put to the test in studies. Let's take a look at some
of those studies—and see why glucosamine passed
with flying colors.

◇ An early, significant study looked at 80 patients in Milan, Italy, all suffering from severe, es-

———————◇———————

Double-blind studies are viewed as the least biased, hence the most preferable, of all the scientific human studies. Since no one knows who is getting the placebo ("sugar" pill) and who is receiving the "real thing," the outcomes are not influenced by hope.

———————◇———————

tablished osteoarthritis.[5] During the course of this 30-day double-blind study, the participants were given either 1.5 grams of glucosamine sulfate or a placebo (a "sugar" pill without any medicinal value). Neither the patients nor the people giving out the pills knew which were the real ones and which were the placebos. (This is what's called a double-blind placebo controlled study.)

Every week, the researchers took measurements of the patients' pain, joint tenderness, and swelling, as well as any restriction of active or passive movement. The final results were positive and exciting:

- The group treated with glucosamine experienced a significantly greater reduction in overall symptoms, compared to those who took the placebo (73 percent versus 41 percent).
- It took only 20 days to reduce the symptoms by half in the glucosamine group, compared to 36 days for those who received the placebo.
- A full 20 percent of the glucosamine-treated

group became completely symptom-free, compared to none of the 40 patients on the placebo!

The impressive results are summed up in this table:

	Glucosamine Group	Placebo Group
No more pain and tenderness	10 out of the 40	0 out of the 40
No more restriction of active and passive movement	9 out of the 40	0 out of the 40
No more overall symptoms	8 out of the 40	0 out of the 40

When the physicians participating in the study were asked to rate the results, they reported that 29 out of the 40 glucosamine patients enjoyed "excellent" or "good" results, compared to only 17 of the 40 who received the placebo. Furthermore, when cartilage samples from the glucosamine-treated patients were examined under an electron microscope, they looked *strikingly similar to healthy cartilage*. But samples taken from the placebo group showed typical evidence of osteoarthritis. In other words, their cartilage looked "sick." The researchers concluded that glucosamine sulfate *rebuilt damaged cartilage*, thereby restoring function in most of the osteoarthritic patients taking the supplement.

◇ And this is only part of the exciting news about glucosamine. Another early double-blind glucosamine study from the Philippines involved 20 patients with osteoarthritis of the knee. Ten patients were given 500 mg of glucosamine 3 times a day while the other 10 received a placebo 3 times a day. Within 6 to 8 weeks, the glucosamine group enjoyed significant reductions in pain, joint tenderness, and swelling, compared to the placebo group. About 80 to 100 percent of the patients taking glucosamine improved during the study, versus only 20 to 40 percent of the placebo group. And no side effects were reported.[6]

Here are the final scores for pain, tenderness, and swelling. The results are presented on a scale of 0 to 4, with 4 being most severe.

Symptom	Glucosamine Group	Placebo Group
Pain	1.25	2.30
Joint tenderness	1.21	2.20
Joint swelling	1.25	2.20

◇ As you can see, the glucosamine group scored lower, which is better, in all three categories. Not only that, the average glucosamine patient showed clinical improvement in approximately 14 days, compared to more than 40 days for the average placebo patient. So impressed were they by the results, the physicians participating in the study concluded that glucosamine sulfate was the first choice for treating patients with osteoarthritis.

―――――――――◇―――――――――

Glucosamine is nontoxic, even at doses that far exceed normal use.

―――――――――◇―――――――――

A study done at the Department of Orthopedic Surgery at Mahidol University in Bangkok, Thailand, also analyzed the effects of injectable glucosamine sulfate versus a placebo in patients with osteoarthritis of the knee.[7] Sixty patients participated in the study, with 30 receiving glucosamine sulfate injections and 30 receiving injections of a saline placebo. The active phase of the study lasted 5 weeks, with 4 weeks of follow-up. Once again, the results were impressive. Thirteen of the glucosamine group became completely pain-free, but only 2 in the placebo group enjoyed a complete remission of symptoms. And on a scale of 1 to 10, with 10 being the most severe, the overall-pain scores were 1.14 for glucosamine patients compared to 6.71 for placebo patients.

Not only were the overall-pain scores lower in the glucosamine group, so were the individual symptom scores. The scores for joint tenderness, pain on standing, pain on walking, and spontaneous pain were rated on a scale of 0 to 3, with 3 being most severe. As you can see, the glucosamine group fared much better (lower scores).

◇ Researchers in Venice, Italy, looked into the effects of injectable glucosamine followed by oral

Symptom	Glucosamine Group	Placebo Group
Joint tenderness	0.29	1.71
Pain on standing	0.36	1.36
Pain on walking	0.50	1.89
Spontaneous pain	0.18	1.61

glucosamine.[8] Thirty patients were randomly assigned to two groups. One group received seven days of glucosamine injections, followed by two weeks of oral therapy of 1.5 grams of glucosamine per day. The second group was injected with piperazine, an Italian anti-arthritic drug, for seven days, then given a placebo-pill for two weeks. Neither the patients nor the doctors who studied them knew which they were getting or giving, so there was no bias in this double-blind study.

The extent of the patients' distress was scored in five areas: pain at rest, pain on active movement, pain on passive movement, restriction of function, and time necessary to walk a certain distance. The results were significant. During the three-week treatment period, the overall-symptom scores for the glucosamine group, on a scale of 1 to 10, dropped from 7.5 to 1.5—and 27 percent of the glucosamine group had no symptoms at all (receiving a 0 on the symptom score). There was no such significant improvement in the placebo group.

The individual results for pain at rest, on active

Symptom	Glucosamine Group	Placebo Group
Pain at rest	0.21	1.13
Pain on active movement	0.67	1.86
Pain on passive movement	0.20	1.07
Restricted function	0.38	1.71

and passive movement, and for restriction of joint function were also measured on a scale of 0 to 3, with 3 being most severe. Again the results were impressive, with the glucosamine scoring much lower (better) in every category.

The glucosamine group was also able to cover ground better: it took them only 29 seconds to walk 20 meters, compared to 50 seconds for those who received the placebo.

In addition to demonstrating how well glucosamine worked, this study showed it to be a mild substance. Most of the patients in this study were severely ill, suffering from circulatory and liver disorders, diabetes, and lung disorders. Some of them were already taking antidepressants and antibiotics. Despite the fact that this was not a healthy group, they all tolerated the glucosamine well, indicating that it is a safe and gentle substance.

◇ A large-scale Portuguese study enlisted 252 doctors in an attempt to see how effectively glucosamine treated osteoarthritis, and how well it would be tolerated by patients.[9] A total of 1,208 patients completed the study and were given 3 daily doses, totaling 1.5 grams of glucosamine, over a period of 36 to 64 days (with an average of 50 days). Their pain was measured four different ways: at rest, while standing, while exercising, and during limited passive and active movements. The results of this study highlight glucosamine's powerful effects:

- Pain improved on a steady basis throughout the treatment period.
- *Ninety-five percent* of the patients in the study enjoyed a "sufficient" or "good" clinical response.
- Glucosamine proved itself to be a long-lasting remedy, continuing to work 6 to 12 weeks *after* the treatment had stopped.
- Eighty-six percent of the patients reported no side effects. (This is a wonderful score, better than you'll find with any drug treatment.)
- Of the small number who experienced side effects, gastrointestinal discomfort was the chief complaint. However, the side effects disappeared on average within 1 to 3 weeks.

On a scale of 1 to 10, with 10 being most severe, overall symptoms for the glucosamine treatment were reduced from a score of 8.7 to 2.5 on average.

In addition to the overall rating, symptoms were measured in specific categories. Here are the pain scores for both groups, presented on a scale of 0 to 3. Patients who had no pain were given a 0. Those with tenderness were given a 1, those who were tender and winced were given a 2, while those who were tender, winced, and withdrew were given a 3. The average scores before and after treatment clearly showed the benefits of glucosamine:

Symptom	Glucosamine-Treated Group	Pre-Treatment Group
Pain at rest	0.3	1.5
Pain on standing	0.5	1.9
Pain on exercise	0.8	2.4

The patients' mobility was also rated on a scale of 0 to 3, with 0 = less than 10 percent hindrance, 1 = 10 to 25 percent hindrance, 2 = 25 to 50 percent hindrance, and 3 = more than 50 percent hindrance. As you can see, glucosamine helped the osteoarthritis patients get moving again.

	Glucosamine-Treated Group	Pre-Treatment Group
Active movements	0.6	1.3
Passive movements	0.4	1.3

◇ Glucosamine has certainly shown its value in a number of studies. But how does it compare to popular pain remedies? Researchers in Portugal pitted glucosamine sulfate against ibuprofen (also known by the brand names Advil, Motrin, Nuprin, and others) in patients with osteoarthritis of the knee.[10] In this double-blind study, 40 patients were given a total of either 1.5 grams of glucosamine sulfate or 1.2 grams of ibuprofen daily (the same as taking 6 over-the-counter pills) over an 8-week period.

The pain levels dropped significantly in both groups during the first two weeks; in fact, the ibuprofen group enjoyed even quicker pain relief than the glucosamine group did. But after the first two weeks the ibuprofen seemed to lose some of its strength, and the pain relief began to fade. Glucosamine, on the other hand, continued strong throughout the treatment period. At the end of the eight-week period there was a dramatic difference in the pain scores between the groups. On a scale of 0 to 3, with 3 being most painful, the glucosamine group had a pain score of only 0.8, compared to the ibuprofen group's 2.2. Additionally, swelling of the knee stopped in 20 percent of the patients in the glucosamine group, compared to none in the ibuprofen group. Overall, 29 percent *more* patients in the glucosamine group had a good outcome.

◇ Glucosamine was also pitted against ibuprofen by scientists from four laboratories, three German and one Italian.[11] Once again, glucosamine sulfate proved to be as effective as ibuprofen in controlling pain—and was much better tolerated. Of the 100 patients in the ibuprofen group, 35 complained of adverse effects throughout the treatment, with 7 dropping out of the study altogether. But only 6 of the 100 patients in the glucosamine group experienced adverse effects, and only 1 dropped out.

◇ Finally, a 30-subject study conducted in Parma, Italy, compared the effects of glucosamine sulfate injections followed by oral glucosamine with a placebo.[12] During a 3-week period, 15 patients received both injections and oral doses of glucosamine, while another 15 received a placebo.

Overall symptoms scores, on a scale of 1 to 10 with 10 being most severe, were rated as 2.4 for the glucosamine group and 8.3 for the placebo group.

Individual symptoms were also assessed. They were rated on a scale of 0 to 3, with 3 being most severe. The results were excellent (low) for the glucosamine group:

Symptom	Glucosamine Group	Placebo Group
Pain at rest	0.33	1.80
Pain upon active movement	0.73	2.20
Pain upon passive movement	0.66	2.13
Function limitation	0.66	2.06

The practical studies bear out the theory—glucosamine *is* a safe and effective treatment for osteoarthritis. By helping the body repair damage to eroded cartilage, glucosamine helps quell pain and relieve swelling and tenderness, with minimal or no side effects.

And it's not just those lucky enough to participate in university studies who enjoy the benefits of
glucosamine. Many individuals are delighted at
their arthritis relief upon taking the supplement.
Sixty-two-year-old Edna Taylor enjoyed being active. After working as a part-time church volunteer
every weekday morning, the cheerful woman
tended her large garden and strolled in the after-
noon. While getting into her car one evening, she
noticed a small "twinge" in her right hip. "It was
nothing," she explained later. "Just like someone
gently pinched me."

A week later, the "gentle pinch" felt more like a
vise grip clamping down on her right hip and upper leg. "When I walked, or even moved my leg, it
felt like someone was hitting me there with a ham-
mer! I couldn't do anything," she said. "No gardening, no walking. Just getting out of the chair to
go to the bathroom was torture. I was really angry.
Why did I get this? And why couldn't the doctors
do anything?"

Not only did she have the original pain, she also
suffered from headaches, blurred vision, and liver
damage, all side effects of the various drugs her
doctors prescribed. "Life used to be fun," she said
dejectedly. "Now it's hell."

Fortunately, the situation improved when Edna
began taking glucosamine. "I didn't notice anything for the first week. I thought it wasn't going
to work and I decided to stop taking it at the end
of Day 9. But when I woke up on Day 10, my hip
felt a little better. So I kept taking it. On Day 15 it

was 25 percent better, and on Day 20 it was 50 percent better. I called my sister to tell her it was 50 percent better, and she didn't believe me."

After taking the supplement for several weeks she was able to tend to her garden and stroll around the neighborhood as much as she had before. And she no longer had to worry about the powerful side effects of standard pain medications.

Don Summers, a 43-year-old world-class bicyclist, came to my office because he was experiencing constant pain and swelling in his knee when bicycling. Despite reconstructive ligament surgery, his knee just never seemed right. Anti-inflammatory medicines and applications of ice weren't working and, unable to exercise and train, Don became very depressed. But within a few weeks of taking glucosamine and chondroitin sulfates, Don really noticed a difference. Today he is 100 percent cured—there is absolutely no pain or swelling. In fact, he showed off his newfound health by giving me a piggyback ride as he jogged down two flights of stairs!

Glucosamine, standing alone, is a fabulous tool for relieving arthritis symptoms and restoring cartilage health. But the relief it brings is further enhanced by the use of a second nutritional supplement—chondroitin sulfates.

The "Water Magnet"

Where glucosamine helps to form the proteoglycans that sit within the spaces in the cartilage "netting," chondroitin sulfates act like "liquid magnets." A long chain of repeating sugars, chondroitin helps attract fluid into the proteoglycan molecules, which is important for two reasons:

- The fluid acts as a spongy shock absorber.
- The fluid sweeps nutrients into the cartilage. Articular (joint) cartilage has no blood supply, so all of its nourishment and lubrication comes from the liquid that ebbs and flows as pressure to the joint is applied and released. Without this fluid, cartilage would become malnourished, drier, thinner, and more fragile.[13]

How does chondroitin ensure that the proteoglycans will attract and hold water in the cartilage? It has to do with chondroitin sulfate "chains." Imagine the tall, strong trunk of a tree stretching into the sky. This is the "backbone" of a proteoglycan molecule. Jutting out from this trunk are large branches (core proteins), and growing from each branch are 100 smaller branches (chondroitin sulfate chains). These chondroitin sulfate chains have negative electrical charges, which means they repel each other. Think of placing two magnets next to each other. If you align them with the opposite poles facing each other, the magnets attract. But if you align them with the same poles facing each other, they repel: The magnets don't want to be pushed together. The negative charges of chondroitin work the same way, pushing chondroitins apart, thus creating a space that forms the matrix of the cartilage. There may be as many as 10,000 of these chains in just a single proteoglycan molecule, making it a super water retainer!

You're already getting some chondroitin sulfates from your diet. Chondroitins are found in most animal tissues, especially in the "gristle" around joints. Some of the chondroitins we eat are absorbed into our bodies intact and incorporated into various tissues, including articular cartilage.

Besides drawing in precious fluid, chondroitin:

- Protects existing cartilage from premature breakdown by inhibiting the action of certain "cartilage-chewing" enzymes.[14]
- Interferes with other enzymes that attempt to "starve" cartilage by cutting off the transport of nutrients.[15]
- Stimulates the production of proteoglycans, glycosaminoglycans, and collagen, the cartilage matrix molecules that serve as building blocks for healthy new cartilage.[16]
- Works synergystically with glucosamine.

Fortunately, supplemental chondroitin sulfates work very much like the naturally occurring chondroitin sulfates in your cartilage, protecting the old cartilage from premature breakdown and stimulating the synthesis of new cartilage. Chondroitin sulfates are nontoxic. A six-year study tracking people taking doses of 1.5 to 10 grams per day has shown no toxicity. This means that we needn't suffer when our natural "healthy cartilage" mechanisms break down. We can replace what the body fails to make.

The "Water Cure" Works!

Just like glucosamine, chondroitin sulfates were put to the test in hospitals and research centers. The results have been surprisingly positive and encouraging.

◊ In 1974, researchers injected chondroitin into 28 patients with severely restricted movement due to osteoarthritis. The injections were given over a period of 3 to 8 weeks. Of the 28 patients 19 exhibited "excellent" results, feeling only slight discomfort when moving and showing no noticeable disability. Six patients showed a significant reduction in pain and could move about more easily. And the average patient continued to experience relief from osteoarthritis symptoms for 7 months after the last chondroitin injection was received.[17]

◊ At the University of Genoa, Italy, researchers compared the effects of injections of chondroitin to a placebo in a double-blind study.[18] The patients, aged 60 to 65, suffered from osteoarthritis of the knee. They were randomly placed into 2 groups of 20. One group received injections of chondroitin sulfate, the other injections of a placebo. All patients also received a nonsteroidal anti-inflammatory drug (NSAID) with each injection. Patients who had used "chondroprotective" agents or corticosteroids during the previous 6 months were not allowed to participate.

The injections were given twice a week for 12 months, and the patients were examined on Days 1, 90, 180, 240, 330, and 360. During the examinations, the patients were evaluated for spontaneous pain, pain on loading, pain on passive movement, pain on pressure, changes in NSAID dose, and side effects. The chondroitin group had a slower rate of pain improvement, but the improvement continued to build during the course of therapy. At the end of the study they had considerably less pain than the placebo group, even though they received gradually *fewer* NSAIDs, while the placebo group did not.

◊ In a particularly interesting study done in France in 1986, 50 patients suffering from osteoarthritis of the knee were given oral doses of either 800 to 1,200 milligrams of chondroitin sulfates, or 500 milligrams of a pain medication.[19] Cartilage tissue samples taken at the beginning of the study and after 3 months of therapy showed that the damaged cartilage in the chondroitin group had repaired itself to a significant degree.

◊ The effects of oral and injectable chondroitin sulfates on elderly people with cartilage degeneration were examined at the University of Naples in 1991.[20] This six-month study involved 200 patients between the ages of 52 and 75. In order to be included in the study, the patients had to have at least five of the following criteria: radiological evidence of osteoarthritis, a typical clinical history of osteoarthritis, exclusion of other types of arthritis, swelling of at least one joint, reddening of at least one joint, hypersensitivity to pressure of at least one joint, and pain when resting or moving of at least one joint.

The patients received either 1,200 milligrams of oral chondroitin sulfate or a 100-milligram injection of chondroitin sulfate. Positive evidence was apparent in the chondroitin group within two weeks. At the end of the study, the researchers concluded that "the results showed a considerable improvement in both pain and mobility. No relevant side effects were found."

◇ A double-blind, randomized study performed in France in 1992 compared the painkilling effectiveness of chondroitin sulfates to a placebo.[21] For this study, 120 patients with osteoarthritis of the knees and hips were given either oral chondroitin sulfates or a placebo. In addition, all of the patients received the same doses of NSAIDs. At the end of three months, the patients taking chondroitin sulfates showed a significant improvement in pain and pain function. The chondroitin was very well tolerated by all who took it. No patients had to withdraw prematurely from the study. As an added bonus, there was a carryover effect: the patients in the chondroitin sulfates group *continued to experience the benefits* during the two-month post-treatment evaluation phase of the study.

◇ Another double-blind, randomized study, this one performed in Buenos Aires, Argentina, in 1987, compared the effects of chondroitin sulfates to those of a placebo.[22] In this study, 34 patients with severe knee osteoarthritis were divided into two groups of 17 each. One group received a daily injection of 150 milligrams of chondroitin sulfates plus 500 milligrams of aspirin three times a day for 20 weeks. The second group was injected daily with a placebo and given the same amount of aspirin. After 20 weeks, 13 of the 17 receiving chondroitin injections experienced an improvement in pain, while only 2 of the 17 in the placebo group enjoyed pain relief—a significant difference.

Glucosamine and Chondroitin Sulfates: The One-Two Punch

Something apparently goes wrong with the cartilage matrix in a person with osteoarthritis. The body doesn't produce proteoglycans and collagen, the building blocks of cartilage, fast enough to keep the cartilage healthy. (This is one of the effects that aging has on cartilage.) At the same time, "cartilage-chewing" enzymes are hard at work, destroying the working cartilage that is present. It's a two-fold problem that needs a two-part solution: glucosamine and chondroitin sulfates.

———————◇———————

*Used together, glucosamine and chondroitin
sulfates enhance cartilage repair and improve
joint function.*

———————◇———————

Working together synergistically, glucosamine
and chondroitin sulfates stimulate the synthesis of
new cartilage while simultaneously keeping the
cartilage-busting enzymes under control. This helps
to normalize the cartilage matrix, in essence treating *the disease at the cellular level*. Other arthritis
treatments relieve pain or reduce inflammation. But
the one-two punch of glucosamine and chondroitin
sulfates can actually halt the disease process in its
tracks and help the body heal itself.

By itself, each supplement is effective. Together,
they may well be the answer for millions of people
suffering from osteoarthritis, the solution that
works where drugs and surgeries have failed. The
combined effects of glucosamine and chondroitin
are being examined in several clinical studies
scheduled to be completed by the end of 1996 or
early 1997. We don't yet have the results of those
studies, but several scientific articles have been
written to explain why these substances work better when taken together. To put it briefly, in order
to qualify as a truly chondroprotective agent, a
compound must be able to:[23]

1. Enhance cartilage cell macromolecule synthesis
   (glycosaminoglycans, proteoglycans, collagens,
   proteins, RNA, and DNA).

2. Enhance the synthesis of hyaluronan (the substance that gives the joint fluid its thick viscosity, providing lubrication between the synovial membrane and cartilage).

3. Inhibit the enzymes that degrade the cartilage cell macromolecules.

4. Mobilize thrombi, fibrin, lipids, cholesterol deposits in synovial spaces, and blood vessels in surrounding joints.

5. Reduce joint pain.

6. Reduce synovitis.

No drug or supplement acting alone can do all that. But glucosamine and chondroitin working together can and do. Clinical studies have shown that glucosamine can accomplish objectives 1, 2, 5, and 6, while chondroitin handles numbers 1, 3, 4, 5, and 6. Their overlapping abilities explain why the glucosamine and chondroitin combination is such a powerful one-two punch against osteoarthritis.

A 42-year-old attorney named Paul Baer found his answer in the combination of glucosamine and chondroitin sulfates. "I used to be a nice attorney," he said laughingly. "I never argued with the other attorneys, I never gave anyone a rough time. I was the opposite of the 'mean attorney' stereotype. Then this arthritis thing hit me in the shoulder. I became the meanest, rottenest guy you ever met, the picture-perfect hateful attorney. And it didn't help that the pills my doctor wanted me to take gave me headaches and stomach problems. I went to another doctor, who recommended glucosamine and chondroitin. The doctor prescribed 1,500 milligrams of each per day, but I'm a cautious guy, so I only took 1,000 milligrams per day the first couple days. Even on that small dose, though, the pain started to go away the very next day. I never even took the full dose, but the pain is completely gone and I'm a nice guy again! You know, I'm lucky. Some of my friends really suffered from their arthritis treatments—even more so than from the arthritis. But the glucosamine and chondroitin cleared up my pain without any side effects."

Celeste Nelson, a 75-year-old widow, prided herself on staying in good shape by walking to the YWCA every morning to do water aerobics, then strolling to the grocery store to do a little shopping. But one day, while carrying two bags of groceries home, Celeste tripped on a raised area of the sidewalk, twisted her ankle, and fell flat on her face, sending apples and oranges flying. There was no one that she could call to come pick her up, so she left the groceries on the sidewalk and slowly hobbled home. The ankle healed completely after several weeks, but the fall must have seriously wrenched her right hip, because pain settled there, refusing to go away. And it slowly grew worse. Even when her ankle healed, the hip pain made it impossible to walk to the YWCA or grocery store anymore.

Celeste heard about glucosamine and chondroitin sulfates from her daughter, a nurse who worked for a nutritionally minded doctor in Beverly Hills. She started taking 1,000 milligrams each of chondroitin and glucosamine and began to feel somewhat better right away. Within five weeks she was able to take walks around the neighborhood. Several weeks after that, she was back to walking to the YWCA for her water aerobics classes. "I'm so glad I can get around. It's a terrible thing for an older person like me to be stuck in the house and dependent on others. Now I'm back to my old self."

A 32-year-old former college football player nicknamed "Buck" had been suffering from pain in both knees ever since "those couple hundred times I was tackled by 250-pound linebackers." Buck described his problem, and the solution: "Knee pain is really incapacitating. You certainly can't run anymore. Walking can be painful, but standing still is really the worst. I can't stand in line at all. If we go to the movies, my girlfriend gets in line for the tickets and popcorn while I sit wherever I can park my rear. If we go to the museum, I either have to rush through it or sit down in front of each exhibit, because I can't stand still; it kills my knees. One of my old football buddies told me about glucosamine and chondroitin. I'm a big guy, so I took 2,000 milligrams of each every day. I didn't expect much because none of the medicines the doctor gave me helped. But it's been about five weeks now, and the pain is halfway gone. I hope the other half goes, too."

If Glucosamine and Chondroitin Sulfates Are So Good...

The theory is sound and the studies are good. So why aren't more doctors using glucosamine and chondroitin sulfates? The reason is a complicated mix of medical conservatism, consumer attitudes, and commercial reality. Throughout their four years of medical school, plus several years more of residency and possibly further training, many physicians are taught that drugs and surgery are the "best" ways to treat patients. Some medical students take a course in nutrition, but the bulk of them receive absolutely no nutritional/dietary training at all. That's why so many doctors turn their noses up at the mere mention of glucosamine and chondroitin sulfates—they're not interested because they don't know any better.

Neither are the pharmaceutical companies interested in glucosamine, chondroitin sulfates, or other nutritional supplements. You see, drug companies like to put their money into products they can patent, like drugs. The patent protects their product, allowing them to corner the market and make a lot of money. Since they can't patent supplements, they don't want to work with them. They don't invest money to study the supplements, and they don't flood doctors' offices with free samples or information about the supplements (as they do with their drugs). Nutritional supplements have traditionally been marketed by smaller companies who do not have the large advertising budgets that the drug companies do.

With neither physicians nor the pharmaceutical industry showing much interest in glucosamine or chondroitin, it's no wonder that the public is either uninformed or wary—or both.

Fortunately, all that is beginning to change, for several reasons:

- The American medical community has recently begun to change its position on what causes osteoarthritis. Thanks to new research on the genesis of osteoarthritis, more and more doctors are realizing that the disease is not an inevitable part of growing older. Normal wear-and-tear is not the problem. Instead, problems with the cartilage matrix are to blame—breakdown is exceeding build-up. Armed with this new understanding, physicians are beginning to look for a way to "fix" the matrix.
- With the increasing internationalization of the drug and health food industries, American doctors are learning about the European research into cartilage repair and regeneration.
- There is a greater general awareness of the healing powers of many nutritional supplements. Melatonin is a recent example of a "health food" that is now being taken seriously as an aid in the battle against the ravages of old age and sleeplessness. And melatonin doesn't have nearly the body of evidence to support its use that glucosamine and chondroitin do.

- More and more physicians are becoming aware of the value of glucosamine and chondroitin sulfates. Aided by the Internet and the work of some well-informed, cutting-edge doctors, more physicians are getting the message. A small but growing number are starting to recommend supplements as part of their treatment protocols, without awaiting for official acknowledgment from the medical establishment.

The change is beginning. We believe that in the near future physicians across the country will be prescribing glucosamine and chondroitin sulfates for many of their osteoarthritis patients on a regular basis.

Where Can I Find/Get Glucosamine and Chondroitin Sulfates?

Glucosamine and chondroitin sulfates can be purchased from a variety of sources, including health food stores, pharmacies, and even some grocery stores. But they are marketed under different names, with different strengths and levels of purity. Chondroitin is most often sold in two forms, chondroitin sulfates and mucopolysaccharides. The chondroitin you purchase should be *pharmaceutical grade* to ensure that it is pure and that it contains the appropriate level of the supplement.

Before rushing out to buy glucosamine and chondroitin sulfates, please study the next chapter carefully. You'll hear how much of each to take, and how to use the two supplements as the spearhead of the nine-step Arthritis Cure. And remember: You don't need a prescription for glucosamine or chondroitin sulfates, but as always, you should speak with your physician before beginning to use these two supplements.

4

◇

The Arthritis Cure

The nine-step Arthritis Cure program.

A laboratory analysis of several glucosamine/ chondroitin sulfate products currently on the market.

◇

Dave Johnson, a 32-year-old salesman, was completely disgusted with the results of his two knee surgeries. "All I wanted was to be able to get around like a normal person, without that damn pain. But both surgeries were a real bust—they changed absolutely nothing. In my job in outside sales I'm in and out of the car maybe 10 times a day, hauling my 25-pound case of samples in and out of office buildings. It's pretty demanding physically, even on a good day, but when your knee is killing you, it's a real grind. I was beginning to think about going into some other line of work when my girlfriend showed me a magazine article on glucosamine and chondroitin sulfates. It said someone my weight should take 1,000 to 2,000 milligrams of each per day, so I took 1,500 of each. I did it for my girlfriend; I never thought they would do anything. It took a week before I felt any improvement, but once it started, the improvement curve got better and better. Every day it was a little better; the pain was a little less. I could do a little more. I've been taking them for two months now and I'm getting around fine at work. I'm even playing on a softball team on the weekends."

Glucosamine and chondroitin sulfates can work wonders on your osteoarthritic joints, but they're only the beginning of The Arthritis Cure. Glucosamine and chondrotin sulfates spearhead the patient-tested, nine-step plan that consists of the following:

1. Have a thorough consultation with a physician.
2. Take glucosamine and chondroitin sulfates to repair damaged joints.
3. Improve your biomechanics to counteract stress to your joints.
4. Exercise regularly.
5. Eat a healthful, joint-preserving diet.
6. Maintain your ideal body weight.
7. Fight depression.
8. Use traditional medicine as necessary.
9. Maintain a positive attitude.

I've had a great deal of success with the Arthritis Cure when treating my patients suffering from osteoarthritis of the knees, hips, back, neck, and other joints. It's not a cure-all, it doesn't work for everyone, but it is undoubtedly the single most effective approach to osteoarthritis, with the least potential for harm. Let's take a look at each of the nine steps.

STEP 1 *Have a Thorough Consultation with a Physician*

A great many conditions mimic the symptoms of osteoarthritis, and lots of people who self-diagnose their problem do so incorrectly. This means that they don't receive the right treatment and may suffer needlessly. Bursitis, for example, causes symptoms similar to those of osteoarthritis and can last for years, but is relatively easy to cure. In most cases gout can be controlled if properly diagnosed and treated. So be sure to get an evaluation from either a medical doctor (M.D.) or doctor of osteopathy (D.O.) who specializes in joint problems. Please remember to consult with your doctor before starting this program.

STEP 2 *Take Glucosamine and Chondroitin Sulfates to Repair Damaged Joints*

The two supplements are the heart of the program. Dosages of glucosamine and chondroitin are usually figured according to your body weight. Although some people may need more and others less, the following dosages are usually effective and serve as a good starting point:

If You Weigh . . .	You Should Take . . .
less than 120 pounds	1,000 mg glucosamine plus 800 mg chondroitin sulfates
between 120 and 200 pounds	1,500 mg glucosamine plus 1,200 mg chondroitin sulfates
more than 200 pounds	2,000 mg glucosamine plus 1,600 mg chondroitin sulfates

Your dosage should be adjusted according to your pain and function. Some people have great results right away and quickly drop their initial doses to half or a third of the starting dose. And some stop taking the two supplements completely after they find their pain has gone for good.

For maximum effectiveness, I recommend that my patients divide their glucosamine and chondroitin supplements into 2 to 4 doses, and take them throughout the day with food. They may also be taken without food, although food seems to help propel them down the esophagus.

Vitamin C and the mineral manganese increase the effectiveness of both glucosamine and chondroitin sulfate and have beneficial effects on joint functions, so make sure these are either included in the supplements that you buy, or take them separately.

Manganese, which is important for synthesis of

cartilage components, is also an antioxidant.[1] A deficiency of this mineral, which often goes unnoticed, can itself lead to osteoarthritis. Found in many whole foods such as nuts, beans, oatmeal, beef liver, and dried peaches, manganese is usually lacking in processed foods. Supplementation appears to be safe in doses up to 50 milligrams per day.

Vitamin C serves as an antioxidant that "recharges" other antioxidants.[2] Because it is water soluble, vitamin C is eliminated from the body in just a few hours (even the "time-released" kind), so taking several smaller doses throughout the day is much more effective than taking one large dose. I generally recommend taking between 500 and 4,000 milligrams of vitamin C per day in 2 to 4 divided doses.

Later on in this chapter you'll find a chart that examines several glucosamine/chondroitin sulfate products currently on the market, telling you their costs, their dosages, just what their labels say they contain, and more important, what our lab analysis revealed several samples actually contained.

STEP 3   *Improve Your Biomechanics to Counteract Stress to Your Joints*

Biomechanics is the study of the mechanical forces exerted to the body by movement. Improper alignment or incorrect use of muscles, bones, tendons, ligaments, and joints can cause excessive wear and tear on the body, leading to injury. The importance of biomechanics in treating osteoarthritis can't be overstated: If you don't correct the underlying problems, you can't rid yourself of the disease.

If the wheels on a car are out of alignment, they will wear badly. You wouldn't just slap a patch on the bald spot or go to the expense of getting new tires. Instead, you fix the alignment. That's what biomechanics can do for your joints—fix the alignment. Many patients have enjoyed "miracle cures" by simply changing the way they walk. A young woman named Nancy Ellis had been to three doctors complaining of severe pain in her right ankle. She had given up tennis, but the pain remained. "The X rays showed nothing, but two of the doctors wanted to operate anyway," she explained, disgusted. Her problem was solved when a biomechanical evaluation showed that she wasn't walking properly. Yes, she was getting from place to place and she looked perfectly normal, but she was putting unusual stress on her right knee, ankle, and foot. She spent a few hours learning how to walk properly, was shown which shoes to buy, and within two weeks her pain was gone for good.

Whether you're a serious athlete, just a weekend dabbler, or one who limits your physical activity as much as possible, you may benefit from a biomechanical evaluation, especially if you have any genetic predisposition toward osteoarthritis. An evaluation will tell you how you are using your joints, the type of stress they are subjected to, and whether anything you are doing might contribute to the development of osteoarthritis down the line. By zeroing in on potential problem areas, you can change the way you use the joint now in order to decrease the risk of problems later. Sports medicine physicians, osteopathic manual therapists, and neuromuscular therapists are among the many professionals that evaluate and treat biomechanical problems.

STEP 4 *Exercise Regularly*

Regular, lifelong exercise fends off a host of health problems. It's also a great way to burn calories and lose weight. And, although we used to think that exercise caused arthritis, we now know that regular, proper exercise is an excellent means of helping to keep joints healthy.

The idea that high-impact exercises such as running could "wear out" joints has been disproved.[3] In fact, regular exercise is strong protection against osteoarthritis.[4] When you bear down on a joint, as you do when exercising, the nutrient-rich fluid in the cartilage is squeezed out, just as if the cartilage were a soggy sponge. Then, when you release the pressure this fluid rushes back into the cartilage, both nourishing it and keeping it moist. The continual rushing in and out of fluid is critical to the health of the cartilage. Without it, the cartilage becomes thin, dry, and more susceptible to damage. In addition to keeping the "cartilage sponge" in action, the proper exercises strengthen the structures around a joint, thereby helping to reduce the pressure the joint is subjected to.

Exercise is also a wonderful medicine for existing osteoarthritis. It keeps the nourishing fluid flowing into the afflicted joint, and reduces pressure on the joint by strengthening supporting structures. The right exercises can often reduce pain and increase mobility. And of course exercise is essential to weight control. (See Chapter 6 for more on exercise.)

"Exercise is great!" That's practically John Wolf's "mantra" now that he can dance with his wife again. The 52-year-old and his wife loved to ballroom dance, but had to give it up when his left knee began bothering him. "It's a screwy concept: You move the thing that hurts when you move it so that it will stop hurting. I never thought that using the leg-weight machines at the club would help my knee, but it has. It may be a screwy concept, but it works. I'll exercise forever, if that's what it takes to keep the pain away from my knee."

STEP 5   *Eat a Healthful, Joint-Preserving Diet*

What you eat (or don't eat) can affect your joints. Certain foods can encourage or discourage the joint-busting free radicals,[5] help to increase or decrease inflammation,[6] and stimulate cartilage repair. The healthful diet described in Chapter 7 lays out a complete nutrition program for counter-

acting the effects of osteoarthritis while keeping
your joints—and the rest of your body—healthy.

STEP 6 *Maintain Your Ideal Body Weight*

Excess pounds are bad news for weight-bearing
joints such as the hips and knees. Researchers have
conclusively linked weight gain and obesity to osteoarthritis, specifically of the knee.[7] In a study
done at Chicago's Cook County Hospital, doctors
noticed that obesity was common in osteoarthritis
patients, and that a large percentage of them had
gained weight just before the disease hit.[8] Fifty percent of those with osteoarthritis had been overweight for 3 to 10 years prior to the onset of the
disease.

Keeping your weight under control is a crucial
part of the Arthritis Cure, for some joints must bear
dozens of times the impact of your body weight
during normal everyday activities. (If you gain just
10 pounds, you may be increasing the force certain
joints must bear from 25 up to 100 pounds!) That's
why staying slim is one of the most important
things you can do for the life of your joints, and
that's why you'll find tips for shedding excess
pounds in Chapter 7.

Many patients have found that losing weight is
a "medicine" in and of itself. "I'm more than a little
embarrassed to say that I had become more than a
tad overweight," 57-year-old Ted Moreno, an ac-
countant, admitted. "I lost the weight because I

didn't like not being able to fit into seats at the movies and on airplanes, but if I had known that dropping the weight would kill that pain in my knees that tortured me for 10 years, I would have gone on a diet years ago! When I think of all the pain pills I took but didn't have to, I'm more than a little annoyed."

STEP 7 *Fight Depression*

It's easy to slide into depression when you can't move without pain, when everything you do seems to be a gigantic effort, and when you feel so *old* all the time. But depression can worsen your pain and interfere with your recovery, so it's vital to begin smiling again as soon as possible. In Chapter 8 you'll learn how to handle the psychological aspects of osteoarthritis, and how positive thinking can energize you as it sets you on the road to recovery.

STEP 8 *Use Traditional Medicines as Necessary*

Although medicines should be used only as a last resort, they can sometimes be the answer for particularly stubborn cases. But learn exactly what they can and cannot offer by reading about pain pills in Chapter 5.

Surgery may also be a final option for osteoarthritis sufferers who have little or no cartilage left (end-stage cartilage loss). In some cases, surgery can help to relieve pain, increase the joint range of motion, and help one get around more easily. Surgery can also be used to align deformed joints. Even if you are having surgery, however, you can benefit from taking glucosamine and chondroitin. The two supplements can help keep you as functional as possible until the surgery takes place and help with pre-surgery rehab. In some cases, they may even delay the need for surgery.

STEP 9 *Maintain a Positive Attitude*

Your attitude toward your condition can make a huge difference, as it does in every other aspect of life. The new medical science called psychoneuroimmunology has shown that the immune system and other parts of the body respond to negative and positive thoughts. In a landmark study, a researcher at UCLA had actors act out "happy" and "sad" scenes. When the actors were *simply pretending to be happy*, the immune system became a little stronger (as measured by the amount of secretory immunoglobulin A). But when they pretended to be sad, their immune systems grew temporarily weaker.[9]

Staying tuned to the positive is a special kind of medicine that can be of value no matter what disease you may be facing. Here are some suggestions to help keep you on the right psychological track:

1. *Don't obsess about your condition.* Complaining and wondering "Why me?" can sap your energy and prevent you from attacking the problem head on. Focus on your treatment, not on what the disease has done to your life. Keep thinking about how good you are going to feel soon, and how much you're going to love getting around just as you used to. The mind-body link cannot be ignored.

2. *Stay connected to friends and family.* Loneliness is a tremendous risk factor for a multitude of diseases, especially for the elderly. Those who are lonely or isolated don't respond to treatment nearly as well as those who are well-connected to a spouse or life partner, family, friends, and their communities. Stay in touch with family and friends; stay involved with life. Get out as much as possible. If you can't get out, invite your friends to visit you. Even getting a pet can be helpful.

3. *Develop a sense of purpose.* People who turn adversity into a challenge have a better prognosis in the long run. If you're hurting, help others, find creative ways to do things you otherwise wouldn't be able to, and look for a beneficial message in your condition. Situations that most people think are hopeless often lead to good.

The positive is always out there, waiting to be seen and used.

Does the Arthritis Cure Work?

The Arthritis Cure offers new hope to those who have been given only a few treatment options in the past. At the very least, the vast majority of patients with osteoarthritis will get *significant relief and may avoid the harmful effects of many "standard" treatments* offered by the current medical system. Here's how the program worked for some people.

Forty-seven-year-old Kathy Watson began suffering from early-morning pain and stiffness in the fingers of her right hand. "That was okay," she said, "and even when my knuckles started making that cracking sound I wasn't that worried. But then the pain got worse during the next year. That's bad for me, because I'm a typist; I use my fingers all day long. It hurt so much I couldn't type well, and couldn't keep up with my work."

A model patient, Kathy carefully followed the Arthritis Cure. "I'm the kind of person that makes a list of what to do, then sticks to it, one, two, three. I got the diagnosis, I took the glucosamine and chondroitin, exactly the right amount at exactly the right time. I did the exercises, I ate well, I thought positively. I did it all, right down the list. My fingers felt better the day after I started, and in maybe two weeks the pain was gone."

Doug Stephens is a 55-year-old dance teacher who spent his youth dancing on Broadway and in plays that toured the nation, doing TV shows, and, of course, taking ballet and jazz classes every single day. "Dance has always been my life," he says. "I can't imagine doing anything else." But by age 50 Doug began noticing pain in various parts of his body, and by 52 he was forced to give up dancing. "I've got osteoarthritis in my lower spine, both hips, and both knees," he said dejectedly. "I'm in constant pain. Luckily I don't have to dance anymore to make a living—I can teach sitting down. But I really want to get up and just boogie sometimes."

Several doctors had told him that he was too young for joint replacement, and that they had nothing to offer but medications. Doug tried the drugs, but couldn't tolerate the side effects. He tried the Arthritis Cure because "at least it didn't sound like it would hurt." Doug was already slim, he followed a very nutritious diet, and used his body in a biomechanically sound manner. "So I focused on the glucosamine and chondroitin, 1,500 milligrams a day of each, and positive thinking," he says. Three months later, Doug reports complete relief from his pain. "I feel like I went out and got a new body! I've been dancing more with my students as I teach, and I'm actually performing in a community theater program next month."

Sixty-two-year-old Joan Simmons went to aerobic dancing class three times a week and played tennis on Monday and Friday mornings at the club. But when osteoarthritis struck in her right hip, she found herself reluctantly cutting back her activities. "I tried to ignore it for as long as I could," she said. "I'd take extra pain medication before playing tennis or aerobics and then ice my hip immediately afterward. I started to develop an ulcer from the pain medicine, and finally I had to admit that osteoarthritis was getting the better of me. I just didn't know what to do."

After starting the nine-step program, Joan was delighted to see rapid results. She gleefully reported, "My pain started getting better a few days after I started the cure. I did the whole thing, except I didn't get the chondroitin because the drugstore where I shop didn't have it. They ordered it. It's been only four weeks and the pain is 80 percent gone! I'm going full throttle with my exercising again. The drugstore finally got in the chondroitin. I'm going to start taking it to get rid of the other 20 percent of the pain."

Of course, not everyone enjoys such rapid and dramatic improvement. Robin Michaels still has some osteoarthritic pain in her left hip after six months of the program. "It's been a long journey to recovery," the 52-year-old homemaker explains. "Both my mother and sister had hip replacements, so I always thought I would have to have one, too. The doctors wanted me to wait until I was older before giving me a new one, but the pain was unbearable. I couldn't get around anymore. And I was so depressed, I ate all day long. I gained fifty pounds. And those drugs they gave me made everything worse."

Robin has been on the Arthritis Cure for six months now. She still has some pain in her left hip, though not nearly as much. "I can get around pretty well," she reports. "I don't feel so depressed anymore, so I don't eat all day long. I do my exercises three times a week, I walk the biomechanically correct way they showed me, and I keep telling myself to be positive. I've lost 40 pounds, which is great. I'm not 100 percent better yet, but I like this. It's working."

And young people can benefit as well. Greg Ostrom is a 22-year-old college senior who "doesn't do much, just play some softball on the weekends. Otherwise, I've been pretty sedentary since I started college. I spend all my time in class, in the lab, or in the library. Or eating pizza," he says.

For reasons unknown, Greg developed severe pain in his left shoulder. It got to the point where he had to fashion a sling to hold his left arm still when he wasn't using it in the chemistry lab. "The orthopedist wanted to operate, but I tried the Arthritis Cure instead because I didn't want someone cutting up my arm. The pain started to go away in the first week. By the third week I took off my sling, and a few weeks after that threw it away," he says with a smile. "Sure beats surgery."

Kathy, Doug, Joan, Robin, and Greg are just five of the many people from all walks of life, of various ages, suffering from differing pains, who have been helped by the Arthritis Cure. Results are usually seen anywhere from one to six weeks after starting to take glucosamine and chondroitin and following the rest of the program. Many people begin by taking NSAIDs or pain medications with the supplements, then taper off of the medications. It's important to remember, however, that just taking the supplements is not nearly as effective as following the entire nine-step plan. Glucosamine and chondroitin are powerful, but they're only the beginning of the Arthritis Cure.

Laboratory Analysis of Glucosamine and Chondroitin Sulfate Supplements

Now that you're ready to begin, you have one more task: finding the right glucosamine and chondroitin sulfates. The labels of supplement bottles all look enticing, but not all products are created equally—and not all are a good buy. Some deliver on the promise, while others could stand some improvement. We've purchased several different products—glucosamine, chondroitin sulfates, and glucosamine/chondroitin combinations—and analyzed them to see how they compare to one another.

The analysis was conducted by the Pharmacokinetics-Biopharmaceutics Laboratory of the University of Maryland at Baltimore (UMAB) under the direction of James Leslie, Ph.D., Research Associate Professor, and Natalie Eddington, Ph.D., Associate Professor. In addition to conducting major laboratory studies, both are professors in the Department of Pharmaceutical Sciences. This independent university research lab performs analyses for a variety of governmental agencies, including the National Institutes of Health, the Food and Drug Administration, and the Environmental Protection Agency, as well as a host of pharmaceutical industry-related

COMBINATION PRODUCTS

	Company Name, Location & Telephone	Supplement Form	Amount of Glucosamine per Capsule/Tablet	Amount of Chondroitin per Capsule/Tablet	Capsules/Tablets Needed for Daily Dosage (per Label)	Price per Bottle	Number of Capsules/Tablets per Bottle
Cosamin DS	Nutramax, Baltimore, MD (800) 925-5187	Capsule	500 mg glucosamine chlorhydrate	400 mg chondroitin	3	$57.00	90
Joint Fuel	TwinLab Ronkonkoma, NY (800) 645-5626	Capsule	250 mg glucosamine sulfate	17 mg chondroitin	6	$25.95	60

GLUCOSAMINE PRODUCTS

	Company Name, Location & Telephone	Supplement Form	Amount of Glucosamine per Capsule/Tablet	Capsules/Tablets Needed for Daily Dosage (per Label)	Price per Bottle	Number of Capsules/Tablets per Bottle
Arth-X Plus	Trace Minerals Research Ogden, UT (800) 624-7145	Tablet	87 mg glucosamine sulfate	6	$21.39	90
Enhanced Glucosamine Sulfate	General Nutrition Corp. Pittsburg, PA (412) 288-4600	Capsule	375 mg D-glucosamine sulfate	4	$19.99	60
Flexi-Factors	Country Life Hauppauge, NY (800) 851-2200 [east] (800) 645-5768	Tablet	63 mg n-acetyl glucosamine 63 mg glucosamine sulfate	3	$16.50	50
Glucosamine Complex	Vitamin Research Products Carson City, NV (800) 877-2447	Capsule	250 mg glucosamine hydrochloride 250 mg n-acetyl glucosamine sulfate	3	$28.95	90
Glucosamine Mega 1000	Jarrow Formulas Los Angeles, CA (800) 726-0886	Tablet	1,000 mg glucosamine hydrochloride	1 or 2	$22.49	100
Glucosamine Sulfate	TwinLab Ronkonkoma, NY (800) 645-5626	Capsule	750 mg glucosamine	2	$44.96	90

Product Name	Company Name, Location & Telephone	Supplement Form	Amount per Capsule/Tablet	Capsules/Tablets Needed for Daily Dosage (per Label)	Price per Bottle	Number of Capsules/Tablets per Bottle
Glucosamine Sulfate	Great Earth Ontario, CA (800) 284-8243	Capsule	500 mg glucosamine sulfate	1 to 3	$13.99	60
Glucosamine Sulfate 500 (Jarrow Formula)	Jarrow Formulas Los Angeles, CA (800) 726-0886	Capsule	500 mg glucosamine sulfate	1 to 4	$27.95	100
Glucosamine Sulfate 500 (The Vitamin Shoppe)	The Vitamin Shoppe North Bergen, NJ (800) 223-1216	Capsule	500 mg glucosamine sulfate with potassium chloride	3	$15.95	60
Joint Factors	TwinLab Ronkonkoma, NY (800) 645-5626	Capsule	375 mg glucosamine	4	$19.96	60
Nutri-Joint	Vitamin Research Products Carson City, NV (800) 877-2447	Capsule	300 mg glucosamine hydrochloride 100 mg n-acetyl glucosamine	3	$38.95	90
Tyler Glucosamine Sulfate	Tyler Encapsulations Gresham, OR (800) 869-9705	Capsule	500 mg glucosamine sulfate	3	$38.00	120
Ultra Maximum Strength Glucosamine Sulfate	Nature's Plus Melville, NY (800) 645-9500	Tablet	600 mg glucosamine sulfate	3	$24.95	60

CHONDROITIN PRODUCTS

	Company Name, Location & Telephone	Supplement Form	Amount of Chondroitin per Capsule/Tablet	Capsules/Tablets Needed for Daily Dosage (per Label)	Price per Bottle	Number of Capsules/Tablets per Bottle
100% CSA (Chondroitin Sulfate A)	TwinLab Ronkonkoma, NY (800) 645-5626	Capsule	250 mg chondroitin	1	$23.95	60
Chondroitin-4 Sulphate	Cardiovascular Research, Inc. Concord, CA (800) 888-4585	Capsule	250 mg chondroitin	2	$16.00	60
Purified Chondroitin Sulfates	American Biologics Chula Vista, CA (800) 227-4458	Capsule	300 mg chondroitin	1 to 3	$33.90	60

companies. This lab and its technicians are highly experienced, with its practices carefully regulated by federal, state, and other national and industry standards.

The laboratory analysis was conducted using standard scientific practices and procedures. Three capsules or tablets from one batch of each product were analyzed to ensure that the results were consistent. The analysis sought to measure the amount of glucosamine or chondroitin actually present in each sample. We were unable to test for the amount of n-acetyl glucosamine.

The charts that begin on this page present some of the samples gathered from across the United States that were analyzed by the UMAB laboratory. All of the samples were found either in health food stores or drugstores. Of those products that we tested, we were surprised to find that in a few instances the amount of either glucosamine or chondroitin found by the laboratory to be present in the sample varied significantly from the amount reported on the label. We have included in these charts only products that UMAB's analysis showed to have essentially what their labels claimed. The charts give you detailed information about each product, including:

- Name and location of the manufacturer.
- The form the supplement comes in—tablet or capsule.
- How many capsules/tablets are needed for one dose.

- The milligrams of glucosamine and chondroitin per capsule or tablet according to the label.
- The total daily dosage.
- The retail price as of mid-1996.
- The number of capsules or tablets per bottle.

As you review the charts, you'll notice that there are many glucosamine products on the market, but relatively few chondroitin or combined glucosamine/chondroitin products. This is most likely because the early studies were performed on glucosamine, so more manufacturers and consumers know about glucosamine, while relatively few are aware of chondroitin. Several studies testing the combined effectiveness of glucosamine and chondroitin are now being conducted. When the results are announced, there will undoubtedly be more glucosamine/chondroitin combination products on the market.

As you read through the charts, you will also notice that different forms of glucosamine and chondroitin are present in the products. Although the forms of glucosamine (sulfate, hydrochloride, n-acetyl, chlorhydrate, D-glucosamine, and with potassium chloride added) sound different, they are essentially the same. There is no known difference between the functions of the various forms of glucosamine—the body metabolizes the glucosamine all the same. And at this point in time there is no evidence to suggest one form is better than the other.

Meanwhile, it's essential to use *both* glucosamine and chondroitin. If your local pharmacy or health food store doesn't carry chondroitin, ask them to order it for you.

There's the nine-step Arthritis Cure. It won't put an absolute end to osteoarthritis, but it has helped many people overcome the pain and other symptoms of this disabling disease. Glucosamine and chondroitin sulfates have worked wonders, but they're not as fast-acting as aspirin or other painkillers. It usually takes between one and six weeks before the results begin to be seen. But remember: The two supplements are only part of the Arthritis Cure. It works best when you follow the entire program.

5

◇

The Problem with Painkillers

What is a nonsteroidal anti-inflammatory drug (NSAID)?

How do NSAIDs work?

Which NSAIDs are used to treat osteoarthritis?

What are the side effects and risks of using NSAIDs?

Can NSAIDs actually make osteoarthritis worse?

What are analgesics?

What are the side effects and risks of using analgesics?

Can the side effects of analgesics and NSAIDs be reduced?

Can NSAIDs be combined with glucosamine and chondroitin sulfate therapy?

Glucosamine and chondroitin sulfates are the treatment of choice for your osteoarthritis because they directly target the source of the problem, instead of simply masking the symptoms. But there are times when painkillers may be necessary, and odds are your doctor will prescribe some for you. Before swallowing any medication, however, it's important that you understand just what it's supposed to do—and what its side effects may do to you.

Although there are numerous drugs with exotic-sounding names, those prescribed for osteoarthritis generally fall into one of two categories:

- Acetaminophen
- Nonsteroidal anti-inflammatories

You're undoubtedly familiar with acetaminophen sold under trade names such as Tylenol, Datril, and Liquiprin. And you've probably already taken nonsteroidal anti-inflammatories such as aspirin, Advil, Aleve, Excedrin-IB, and Motrin. (Nonsteroidal anti-inflammatory drugs are often called NSAIDs for short, which is pronounced "n-sayds.")

There are major differences between acetaminophen and the NSAIDs, both of which are excellent pain relievers. Acetaminophen is an analgesic and antipyretic, which means that it relieves pain and lowers fever. NSAIDs do a little more: they fight pain, lower fever, *and* reduce inflammation.[1] If you have joint swelling and inflammation your doctor will probably prescribe NSAIDs. If your pain is not accompanied by inflammation, your physician will probably opt for acetaminophen since it's less expensive and has fewer side effects than NSAIDs. Of course, that doesn't mean that acetaminophen doesn't have some side effects of its own.

At a standard or usual dosage level (below 4 grams per 24-hour period), acetaminophen is generally well-tolerated and safe. But when taken over a long period of time, acetaminophen can cause a small but significant decrease in liver function, and it can harm the kidneys.[2] In fact, heavy use of acetaminophen may be the culprit in as many as 5,000 cases of kidney failure each year in the United States. (If you do take acetaminophen, you can reduce your risk of kidney failure by taking it with food and avoiding alcohol.[3])

Acetaminophen plays an important role in osteoarthritis. But if your joints become painful, swollen, and stiff, your doctor will probably look to the NSAIDs.

———————◇———————

*NSAIDs come in several forms—pill, liquid,
injection, and suppository.*

———————◇———————

The NSAID Story

Developed as alternatives to the corticosteroids,
NSAIDs have become a popular choice for physicians treating osteoarthritis. Corticosteroids such
as cortisone and prednisone are sometimes necessary. They are great at reducing pain and inflammation, but they have some nasty side effects that
make them downright dangerous—like depress-
ing the immune system, thinning the bones, increasing the risk of bone fracture, and impairing
wound healing. When taken in high doses for
long periods of time, corticosteroids can cause hypertension, diabetes, osteoporosis, and even mental disturbances.[4] That's why a substitute for the
corticosteroids, such as the NSAIDs, was so necessary—and welcome.

Aspirin is the most popular and best known of
the NSAIDs—in fact, it was being used long before
the concept of NSAIDs was ever dreamed of. In
1758, the Reverend Edward Stone found that an extract from willow tree bark helped reduce fever and
pain in 50 of his patients. The extract was studied
and refined for years, finally emerging as a non-

---◇---

*Aspirin belongs to a family of drugs called
salicylates. The name refers to the active
ingredient in the drug.*

---◇---

steroidal anti-inflammatory that became known as common aspirin.

Other NSAIDs were developed in the 1960s. First was indomethacin (Indocin), and then came ibuprofen (Advil, Motrin).[5] Today, there are more than 100 different NSAIDs either on the market or being investigated. Over-the-counter (nonprescription) NSAIDs include Advil, Aleve, Nuprin, Excedrin-IB, Midol 200, Motrin, and Orudis.

NSAIDs work by blocking the production of prostaglandins, hormonelike substances in the body that "cause" the pain and inflammation responses.[6] But the prostaglandins have many other important and necessary duties, playing a role in the regulation of blood pressure, blood coagulation, kidney regulation, and the secretion of gastric acid. Anything that interferes with the "bad" actions of the prostaglandins will hamper these "good" ones as well. That's why taking continual high doses of the NSAIDs commonly interferes with vital bodily activities, triggering side effects such as:[7]

- nausea
- cramps

- indigestion
- diarrhea
- constipation
- sensitivity to sunlight
- nervousness
- confusion
- drowsiness
- headache
- ulcers or stomach bleeding
- sore throat or fever (these may be early signs of a bone marrow disorder, and are associated with taking phenylbutazone)
- swelling of the fingers, hands, feet; weight gain; urinary problems (these may all be signs of heart or kidney disorders and should be immediately reported to your doctor)
- anaphylaxis (Rare, severe allergic reaction characterized by difficulty in breathing or swallowing, a swollen tongue, dizziness, fainting, hives, puffy eyelids, fast and irregular heartbeat or pulse, or a change in face color. This is an emergency situation; you should immediately seek help if you experience any of these signs.)
- high blood pressure

And there is growing evidence that NSAIDs may inhibit the synthesis of proteoglycans, important molecules that attract water to the cartilage. In other words, the pills we take to block osteoarthritis pain may actually decrease the action of proteoglycans.

When used for short-term relief from pain and inflammation, NSAIDs can be quite helpful. But by quelling pain they can disguise or "mask" your osteoarthritis symptoms. You may believe that your condition is under control because your shoulder feels okay or your knee isn't as swollen. But the disease process *does* continue, whether you feel its effects or not.[8] To make matters worse, some studies have inferred that NSAIDs not only don't delay the progression of osteoarthritis, they may actually *hasten* it.[9]

I have a personal interest in the side effects of NSAIDs. My 93-year-old grandmother had been on various NSAIDs for years due to severe osteoarthritis of her knees. Unfortunately, she developed kidney problems from these drugs. I have taken her off of the drugs and her kidneys are now stable, but I wish I had known about glucosamine and chondroitin sulfates sooner. They work without measurable side effects, even with long-term use.

Determining a Drug's Effectiveness

NSAIDs are grouped according to their "half-lives," or the length of time the drugs are in the body at levels high enough to be therapeutic. You can think of the half-life as a medicine's "effective life." Either an NSAID has a short half-life (less than six hours) or a long one (more than ten hours).[10] Both types, short-acting and long-acting, have advantages and disadvantages:[11]

Short-acting medications are rapidly absorbed into the body, acting quickly on the symptoms. They are also rapidly eliminated from the body, which helps to prevent toxic reactions. But this quick kind of "in and out" action means that the medicines have to be taken more frequently, for their action is short-lived. This can be a problem for people who are busy or forgetful or just plain don't like to take pills.

Long-acting medications can be taken once and forgotten for the rest of the day. This makes them good choices for those who can't or won't take pills every few hours. But these medicines are stronger milligram per milligram and stay in the body longer, which increases the risk of accumulated toxicity. That's why long-acting drugs are not usually prescribed for patients with kidney problems or for some elderly patients, regardless of their overall health. Another disadvantage of the long-acting NSAIDs is that when a patient is experiencing severe pain, he or she may feel helpless while waiting for the minutes or hours to crawl by until the next dosage time.

Here are the most commonly prescribed NSAIDs[12] and their "effective lives" (half-lives):[13]

Generic Name	Brand Name	"Effective Life"[14]
Phenylbutazone*	Butazolidin, Azolid	68 ± 25 hours
Oxyphenbutazone*	Tandearil, Oxalid	58 ± 10 hours
Indomethacin	Indocin, Indocin SR	4.6 ± 0.7 hours
Ibuprofen	Motrin, Rufen	2.1 ± 0.3 hours
Fenoprophen calcium	Nalfon	2.5 ± 0.5 hours
Tolmetin sodium	Tolectin	1.0 ± 0.3; 6.8 ± 1.5 hours†
Naproxen	Naprosyn	14 ± 2 hours
Sulindac	Clinoril	14 ± 8 hours
Meclofenamate sodium	Meclomen	57 ± 22 hours
Piroxicam	Feldene	Is long-acting‡
Salicylsalicylic acid	Disalcid, Mono-Gesic	2–15 hours
Aspirin	Bayer, Bufferin	0.25 ± 0.3 hours
Diflunisal	Dolobid	13 ± 2 hours

*Used specifically in the short-term treatment of osteoarthritis of the hips and knees that are not responsive to other treatment.

†Drug elimination occurs in two phases; the first is the most important.

‡No comparable data available.

Let's take a closer look at these drugs:[15]

Phenylbutazone and oxyphenbutazone have been on the market since 1952 and 1961 respectively. Today, however, their use is highly restricted and controlled, for they may cause two fatal blood diseases called agranulocytosis and aplastic anemia. They have also been shown to cause a lupus-like condition. Phenylbutazone is used as a last resort and only on a short-term basis, but can be effective in treating ankylosing spondylitis, gout, tendinitis, or bursitis. In addition to the side effects mentioned above, it can cause stomach upset, as well as water and salt retention, leading to rapid weight gain. This medication should not be taken with other arthritis drugs, including aspirin.

Indomethacin effectively relieves moderate to severe osteoarthritic pain of the hip, as well as bursitis of the shoulder. This drug's most common side effects include peptic ulcers, gastrointestinal upset, severe headaches, dizziness, rashes, ringing in the ears, and depression. Should depression occur, you will probably be taken off the drug.

Ibuprofen, remarkably similar to aspirin in its anti-inflammatory properties, has been successfully used to treat the symptoms of both osteoarthritis and rheumatoid arthritis. The most common side effects associated with ibuprofen include gastrointestinal problems, nausea and vomiting, dizziness, and skin rash.

Fenoprophen calcium is similar to ibuprofen and naproxen in its chemical makeup. Its side effects include gastrointestinal disturbances, ulcers, dizziness, skin rash, and ringing in the ears. Fenoprophen calcium drugs can interact with several other medications, so care must be taken when prescribing it.

Tolmetin sodium, prescribed primarily to treat symptoms of rheumatoid arthritis, interacts adversely with several other drugs. Tolmetin has also been associated with reversible kidney failure, and at high doses can upset the stomach.

Naproxen is an effective treatment for the symptoms of osteoarthritis, and is usually well-tolerated. Its side effects include gastrointestinal distress, peptic ulcers, dizziness, rash, and occasionally, fluid retention.

Sulindac, which is similar in chemical makeup to indomethacin, is effective in treating the symptoms of osteoarthritis of the hip, knees, and cervical spine, as well as bursitis of the shoulder. It's better tolerated at higher levels than both indomethacin and aspirin, but does have potentially serious side effects such as irritation of the gastrointestinal tract, vertigo, insomnia, sweating, rash, and a rare condition manifested by painful, swollen, discolored toes.

Meclofenamate sodium is an effective treatment for acute and chronic osteoarthritis, as well as rheumatoid arthritis. But meclofenamate is not recommended as a first-line defense because its gastrointestinal side effects (nausea, diarrhea, or stomach pain) can be severe. Alcohol, aspirin, and other arthritis drugs should be avoided when taking this medication.

Piroxicam, a recent addition to the NSAID family, has been successful in treating the symptoms of osteoarthritis, rheumatoid arthritis, gout, and ankylosing spondylitis. It's taken only once a day, which makes it particularly good for forgetful or noncompliant patients. The drug's most common side effects are gastrointestinal distress, plus a rash caused by increased sun sensitivity.

Aspirin and salicylates—Aspirin and the class of drugs to which it belongs, salicylates, have been used for more than 100 years to treat osteoarthritis, rheumatism, and just about any other kind of pain. Derived from the bark of the willow tree, these drugs block the production of prostaglandins, hormonelike substances in the body that can bring about fever, inflammation, and pain. Small doses are used to treat pain, with larger doses prescribed for inflammation. Their prowess in treating the symptoms of osteoarthritis has been well documented. Of course, aspirin and other salicylates have side effects. Patients often stop taking the drugs because of side effects such as gastric intolerance, which can range from minor stomach upsets to life-threatening hemorrhages. Some of the salicylates commonly prescribed for osteoarthritis symptoms are:

- Aspirin (Bayer, Bufferin, Ecotrin)
- Choline magnesium trisalicylate (Trilisate)
- Diflunisal (Dolobid)
- Magnesium salicylate (Magan)
- Salicylsalicylic acid (Disalcid, Mono-Gesic)

Phenylbutazone, naproxen, piroxicam, salicylates and the rest: None of these drugs actually cures osteoarthritis. They may help relieve the pain, swelling, and inflam-

mation, and they may make it easier for you to use your joints, but they are not a cure. And all of them have potentially serious side effects that limit their usefulness. That's why glucosamine and chondroitin sulfates have a "leg up" on the drugs. Glucosamine and chondroitin work at the cellular level to help damaged cartilage heal. They don't simply mask the problem—they work to make it go away.

To be fair, NSAIDs provide faster pain relief than either glucosamine and chondroitin sulfates, but the relief quickly plateaus and often diminishes with time. If your symptoms are severe, you may want to use one of these painkillers for a week or two in conjunction with glucosamine and chondroitin sulfates, then taper off of the medication as the nutritional supplements begin to rebuild the cartilage matrix. Of course, you should check with your physician before beginning or altering any medicinal regimen.

Minimizing the Side Effects

Although side effects are common when taking NSAIDs, these unwelcome visitors can often be turned away by following these guidelines:[16]

- In general, all NSAIDs should be taken with food. It's often helpful to eat, take the pill, then eat again.
- In order to control the development of ulcers while you're taking NSAIDs, your doctor may

prescribe Misoprostol. If you're pregnant, your doctor will suggest a different medication.

- Drink at least eight ounces of water when taking tablets or capsules to keep the lining of the esophagus and stomach from becoming irritated.
- Don't lie down for 30 or so minutes after taking your medicine. Gravity helps assure that the pill passes through the esophagus (food tube).
- Always take the exact dose prescribed by your doctor. Never double it, even if you miss a scheduled dose.
- Pregnant or breast-feeding women should not take NSAIDs unless specifically directed to and monitored by a doctor.
- Do not use alcohol while taking NSAIDs, for doing so increases the risk of stomach problems.
- Don't combine acetaminophen (such as Tylenol) or aspirin with NSAIDs unless specifically directed to do so by your doctor.
- Inform your doctor of all other medications you are taking, whether prescription or over-the-counter, so he or she can determine whether one drug will interact with another.
- If you are having surgery, inform your doctor or dentist that you are on NSAID therapy, even a low dose.
- Avoid driving or operating machinery when you are taking NSAIDs, for they may cause drowsiness, confusion, or dizziness in a small number of patients.
- Be careful in direct sunlight. Your skin's sensitivity may be increased during NSAID therapy.

Before Taking Any Medicines

Drugs are powerful weapons against distress. But they're not "smart bombs" that know exactly what to target. Many, many people have been harmed by medicines that destroyed the wrong target in the body. Physicians are supposed to make sure that patients get exactly the right medicine at the right dose at the right time and for the right reason. Unfortunately, that's not always the case. Sometimes doctors are unaware of a medicine's side effects or forget to ask which drugs you are already taking before prescribing a new one. The situation is getting even worse with the move toward managed care, for now many doctors are pressured or required to prescribe a limited number of drugs, even if another one may be better suited to your needs.

That's why it's up to you to ask questions—plenty of them—before agreeing to take *any* medicine. Insist that your doctor answer all your questions fully. Don't accept "don't worry about it" or "you wouldn't understand" for an answer. Here are some of the questions you should ask:

- Why do I need this drug?
- What are the possible side effects, from the most common to the very least?
- Who is most likely to suffer these side effects?
- What early signs will warn me that the side effects may be striking?
- Is there another medicine better suited to my needs?

- Is there a generic version of the drug that would work just as well for me but costs less?
- How many times a day should I take the medication? When? Should I take it with food or water, or on an empty stomach?
- Are there any foods or drinks I should avoid while taking this drug?
- Are there any activities I should restrict or avoid while taking this drug?
- How soon should the drug begin working?
- How will I know it's working?
- Assuming it works, how long should I continue taking it?
- If it doesn't work, how long before we try something else?
- Is there a nondrug treatment I might try?

After you've questioned your doctor, be sure to tell him or her if you are already taking any other drugs, nutritional supplements, or other substances. And mention whether or not you've had adverse reactions, allergies, or sensitivity reactions to *any* medicines or other substances. Even the smallest reaction may be important, so don't hesitate to speak up.

Remember: Doctors are sometimes quick to prescribe drugs, but every single drug has side effects. You are not required to swallow everything your doctor gives you. Feel free to ask questions. And if you don't like the answers, insist on hearing about other treatment options. *When it comes to your health, you're the boss*. You have the right to have all your questions answered completely and to your satisfaction before you make a decision.

If your doctor prescribes medicines for your osteoarthritis, ask about glucosamine and chondroitin. If your physician is not aware of these two nutritional supplements, show him or her this book.

6

◇

Exercise That *Helps*, Not Hurts

Why is exercise so important?

Can exercise help damaged joints? Or does it actually cause osteoarthritis?

Does it strengthen bones?

Can it really prevent joint deformities?

Which exercises are best?

Why is stretching necessary?

How does exercise reduce my fatigue level?

How do I get started?

A 75-year-old retired high school teacher, Bill had lived an active life, working with teenagers, gardening, camping, backpacking, and acting as the neighborhood "fix it" man. Anytime anyone in the neighborhood had a problem with their sprinklers or their plumbing or their gas heaters, they called on "good ol' Bill," who graciously came over to lend a hand.

Once he turned 70, though, the osteoarthritis that had bothered his left knee for some time started to get pretty bad. Luckily he wasn't teaching anymore—all that standing would have been impossible. And camping and backpacking were pretty much a thing of the past. At first he took these changes in stride. But before long he had to give up gardening and couldn't even walk halfway down the block to help a neighbor. A friend suggested he try water aerobics at the YMCA. He did, and the results were surprising. "Exercising in the water is great because it supports your weight. Since I've been doing it, my knee is a lot less stiff, I don't limp as much and some days it barely hurts at all. I guess exercise is sort of like greasing up a rusty door hinge and then working the grease in by opening and closing the door a bunch of times."

Bill's explanation of why exercise helps ease osteoarthritis symptoms is actually not too far from the truth. It may sound strange, but one of the best medicines for osteoarthritis is exercise. The right kind of exercise can ease your symptoms, help you to lose weight, and help to take a load off your joints. It also improves immune functioning and enhances your overall health. Even aerobic exercise, which is often thought to be too strenuous, can be beneficial to people with osteoarthritis.[1]

For a long time, doctors believed that exercise aggravated or even caused osteoarthritis, and they advised against it. Perhaps that's one reason why very few osteoarthritis sufferers exercise on a regular basis. That's a shame, for they're missing out on a powerful and often fun treatment.

The Importance of Exercise

We have a natural tendency to slow down when we're injured or sick, to stop our normal activities in favor of rest. And that's often the wisest course. But in the case of osteoarthritis, too much sitting around can be devastating. We're designed to be up and around most of the day, walking, stooping, gathering, hunting, or working the fields. Our bodies have built-in mechanisms to conserve energy and prevent starvation. *Atrophy*—the wasting away of unused muscle and bone to lessen energy expenditure—is one of those mechanisms. This happens to osteoarthritis sufferers who cut back drastically on the amount of exercise. They lose strength, tone, and flexibility of their muscles. Joint range of motion becomes limited and the bones thin, while cartilage both thins and softens. When this happens, osteoarthritis progresses more rapidly.

Exercise helps to keep joints healthy. Even

though glucosamine and chondroitin sulfates re-build cartilage while reducing osteoarthritic symptoms, it's very important to continue exercising. Movement in any of its many forms, whether it be walking, running, lifting weights, swimming, and so on, is now widely accepted as an important part of the treatment for osteoarthritis. It fights the debilitating effects of this disease in two major ways:

Exercise encourages the flow of synovial fluid into and out of the cartilage. Synovial fluid lubricates and nourishes cartilage: its very presence is believed to slow the progression of osteoarthritis. The constant movement of liquid into and out of the spongy cartilage keeps the cartilage moist, healthy, and well nourished. But without the pressure created by movement and exercise, the liquid will not flow in and out. Then the cartilage starts to dry out and becomes thin, like an old piece of shoe leather, losing its resilience in the process. Exercise helps to prevent this from happening by keeping joints "wet" and well nourished. (This helps explain why an osteoarthritis sufferer will often have the most discomfort right after a period of inactivity—the joint has not been nourished for a while. The phenomenon is sometimes called "movie goer's knee.")

Exercise strengthens the supporting structures (muscles, tendons, ligaments) and increases the range of motion, shock absorption, and flexibility of the joints. Strong, well-toned muscles, tendons, and ligaments can bear the brunt of the force that crashes into joints as we move, while helping the bones support the body. In fact, the majority of the load that the joints bear can be transferred to these supporting structures, allowing the articular cartilage to maintain its integrity.[2] Exercise also allows us to move better (also known as better biomechanics).

And that's not all. Exercise's many other benefits to mind and body include:

- Improving your physical capabilities.
- Preventing joint deformities.
- Contributing to better emotional health.
- Reducing stress.
- Enhancing sleep.
- Promoting relaxation.
- Improving body composition (that is, gaining muscle, losing fat).
- Increasing your resistance to other diseases.
- Building up a reserve capacity in the event of disease.
- Improving sexual function, satisfaction, and body image.
- Improving balance.
- Helping you preserve your independence.

Lack of regular exercise contributes greatly to the development of high blood pressure, obesity, diabetes, and heart disease. In fact, a sedentary lifestyle is second only to smoking as the most common cause of disease and death in the United States. Even the simplest of exercises can be tremendously helpful. The importance of walking or water aquatics was demonstrated by a study done at the University of Missouri. Of the 120 subjects, 80 had osteoarthritis. The participants were randomly assigned to two groups: one with an exercise program consisting of either aerobic walking or aerobic pool aquatics; the other a control group consisting of nonaerobic range-of-motion exercises. Each group met three times a week for an hour for a total of 12 weeks. The results were impressive. By the end of the study:

- The aerobic group showed significant improvement in aerobic capacity, walk time, and physical activity level after the 12 weeks of exercise.
- Upon comparison to two drug studies, the exercise study participants had at least as good results.[3]

If simple exercises can reduce pain and improve your ability to move, imagine what a full exercise program can do for you.

Exercise Also Strengthens Bones

Bones are not like the pillars holding up bridges or the steel beams inside buildings. The pillars and beams are static—they don't change. But bones are constantly changing. The *osteoclasts* in our bones continually tear down old bone cells, while the *osteoblasts* build new ones. Bones are dynamic, not static, constantly changing in response to the changing demands made upon them. In that sense bones are quite a bit like muscles, growing thicker and stronger in response to a heavier work load. In fact, obese people tend to have very strong bones because they have to support so much weight. (Gaining weight to increase your bone strength is not advised, however.)

Years of study have proven that regular exercise increases bone density, thereby making bones stronger. But not any exercise will do. The two kinds of exercise that help bones grow stronger and thicker are *weight-bearing exercise* and *strength training*.[4]

Weight-bearing exercise is simply related to gravity. This means that your bones have to hold you up, working against the force of gravity. Walking is a weight-bearing exercise for the feet, legs, and hips. Gravity has less and less effect as you move up the spine. For example, your neck has only the weight of your head on it, but your lower back must support the weight of the head, arms, and trunk. And the feet support the weight of everything. Generally, weight-bearing exercises work the lower body more than the upper body. (Although that's not to say that they are useless for the upper body, because it *is* taking on some of the load.)

The second kind of exercise that helps build bones and keep them strong is *strength training*. Also called resistance training, it involves repeatedly lifting or moving a load (weight) to the point of muscle fatigue. Lifting free weights (dumbbells or barbells) and using weight machines and resistance devices like elastic tubing are all examples of strength-training exercises. You don't have to lift hundreds of pounds to improve your strength. For many, 5-to 10-pound weights are all it takes to get started.

If the repetitions (number of times you lift the load) are limited by muscle fatigue to about 15 or less, the exercise is strength training. If you do more than 15 repetitions, the exercise becomes *muscle-endurance training*. Muscle-endurance training has its benefits, but isn't nearly as efficient at improving strength, muscle, and bone mass. If you want to do strength training and you find that you can do more than 15 repetitions of an exercise without muscle fatigue, it's time to increase the amount of weight rather than increasing the number of reps.

All About Exercise and Fitness

One of the primary goals of exercise is to improve fitness. There are seven types of fitness, including:

- strength
- aerobic capacity
- flexibility
- agility/balance
- sport-specific fitness
- power
- speed

Only the first four types are required for health and the prevention of osteoarthritis. Let's take a look at the first four types of fitness in detail:

STRENGTH

Are your legs strong enough to get you out of a chair? Can you easily lift bags of groceries? Can you do a chin up using just your arms? Can you squat on the floor and raise yourself on one leg without help from your hands? You need strength to accomplish these tasks.

Strength is important for shock absorption in the joints, good bone health (prevention of osteoporosis), ambulation (the ability to move), reserve capacity in illness, weight loss, and weight control. It's also important for preventing injuries; for instance, if you're not strong enough to lift something, you may damage yourself while lifting it improperly.

Exercises that improve strength include weight lifting (free weight and machines), rock climbing, heavy manual labor, and any activity that causes your muscles to fatigue after a small number of repetitions.

AEROBIC CAPACITY

Do you get winded walking up a hill? Can you walk a block? A half mile? A mile? After you've walked a long distance, does your heart pound so hard that you feel as if you must stop?

In a very simple sense, your aerobic capacity is your ability to keep moving, even when you're tired. Exercises that increase your aerobic capacity (including your breathing capacity and muscle endurance) have many other benefits, such as improving joint shock absorption and bone health (prevention of osteoporosis), weight control, and preventing stroke and heart disease. Brisk walking, running, biking, swimming, stair climbing, cross-country skiing, rowing, certain forms of dancing, many sports, plus aerobics and step classes can improve your aerobic capacity and cardiovascular fitness. Any activity that gets your heart rate up and can keep it up for at least 15 to 20 minutes consecutively is considered aerobic.

FLEXIBILITY

Can you sit on the floor with your legs together, knees straight, and touch your toes? When you bend down to pick up something, does your back only seem to bend in the lower region? Can you reach any spot that itches on your back?

Good flexibility is vital. Areas of relative inflexibility cause excess stress and force to be exerted on other areas of the body. This can lead to altered biomechanics, overcompensation, and osteoarthritis. And inflexible tissues are more likely to become strained or sprained.

Exercises that can improve your flexibility include yoga, stretching (all kinds), ballet and other forms of dancing, and most of the martial art forms.

Agility/Balance

Do you have difficulty with balance? Do you have to grab on to furniture to steady yourself occasionally? Can you balance yourself while standing on one foot? With your eyes closed?

Good balance and agility allow you to maintain your activities with confidence as you age, and can help to prevent falls. Balance also improves your body's biomechanics by maximizing your ability to distribute shock for more effective absorption.

Exercises that improve agility and balance include yoga, ballet and other forms of dancing, most of the martial art forms, and sports that involve quick changes of direction (such as racquet sports).

Sport-Specific Fitness

Do you have a good-looking golf swing? Is your tennis serve fast, hard, and smooth? Do you say things like "I can walk forever, but my legs really get tired when I ski moguls"?

Sport-specific exercises are very useful for preventing injuries and, by extension, the osteoarthritis that they may induce. If you don't play a particular sport, you needn't worry about sport-specific exercises. But if you do, make sure your body is toned and prepared to play properly. Exercises that improve sport-specific fitness include the sport's drill exercises and playing the actual sport itself. Cross-training activities may help too, such as playing soccer to help with the accuracy of football place-kicking.

POWER AND SPEED

Can you run and jump quickly over a fence? How far can you throw a baseball or hit a golf ball? How fast can you run 50 yards?

Although power and speed are not necessary for modern-day survival, or to prevent osteoarthritis, they are essential for good performance in many sporting activities. Exercises that improve power include power lifting (not just lifting weights but lifting them quickly), football drills, and ballistic activities like plyometric training. Exercises that improve speed include sprinting of all types (whether on foot, on skis, on a bike, on skates, etc.) and specific speed drills.

The Types Are Linked

The fascinating thing about the seven different types of fitness—and the four we're concerned with here—is that generally they are all lost at the same rate as we age and slow our activity levels. Balance, agility, strength, aerobic capacity, and flexibility are all lost by lack of use. Luckily, most kinds of exercise work on more than one area of fitness. For instance, walking can improve aerobic fitness and muscle endurance, while also maintaining and improving balance and agility. Playing a game of ten-

———————◇———————

Range-of-motion exercises can be done in a pool if you have acute joint pain.

———————◇———————

nis may encompass aerobic fitness, agility/balance, flexibility, speed, and power.

Aerobics, Jogging, Lifting, or What?

Even if you already have osteoarthritis and are limited in your ability to move one or more joints, there are many exercises you can do. But before choosing the exercises you want to do, think about your goals. An exercise program for osteoarthritis should do two things: strengthen the supporting structures of the joint and increase the joint's range of motion.

• *Strengthening supporting structures.* There are many ways to strengthen the muscles that work with your joints. Anything that involves lifting strengthens a muscle, from rearranging your closet to weight training. Walking, jogging, bicycling, dancing, and anything else that involves moving the body from place to place is good for the leg muscles. Swimming is an excellent toner for many muscles in the shoulders, back, arms, and legs. If you like walking but would like to give your arms a little workout at the same time, try carrying small weights in your hands or wearing wrist weights.

———————◇———————

It's easy to incorporate exercise into your daily routine. You can park farther away than you normally do and walk, or take the stairs instead of the elevator. Even gardening is exercise.

———————◇———————

And don't forget to consider a very important supporting structure: your heart. A good aerobic workout, the kind that gets your heart beating harder and your breath coming faster, strengthens your heart and circulatory system, allowing you to increase your level of exercise and, therefore, your level of fitness. It also helps you keep your weight under control and can give you an emotional boost.

• *Increasing range of motion.* Just using a joint is a simple way to hold on to whatever range of motion you currently have. But stretching is the best way to *increase* your joints' range of motion. Gentle stretching helps to loosen up the muscles while making the tendons and ligaments more flexible and resilient. This, in turn, means that your joints will move more easily and stiffness will be reduced. Stretching also improves overall joint function, lessens joint pain, and releases pent-up tension. A more relaxed outlook on life and a better night's sleep are two extras that often accompany stretching's better-known benefits. So stretch regularly!

Strengthening, aerobics, balance, and stretching exercises can be performed safely and effectively by most osteoarthritis sufferers. However, *common sense and moderation are always the rules when exercising.* Ask your doctor, exercise physiologist, or physical therapist to tailor an exercise program to your specific needs and limitations. If you have an acute flare-up, your doctor may suggest that you do your exercises in the pool in order to take the weight off your joints, or he or she may ask you to stop exercising altogether for a short period of time. Remember that it's always a good idea to check with your doctor before returning to your normal exercise plan after you've had any problem.

Designing Your Exercise Program

Exercise sounds like a simple matter—put on your sneakers and start sweating. However, finding the right exercises that strengthen your bones and supporting structures can be a little more complicated. Given that you may have already damaged one or more of your joints, strained the supporting structures, and possibly produced muscle imbalances, it would be wise if you began by enlisting the help of your physician, who can determine your general level of fitness and strength. He or she should evaluate your muscle strength, range of motion, and dexterity, as well as your ability to do simple tasks such as walking up and down stairs. The doctor will probably recommend a physical therapist or exercise physiologist, who will devise an exercise program for you based on your doctor's specifica-

---◇---

If you experience discomfort more than an hour after exercising, you've probably overdone it.

---◇---

tions. The physical therapist or physiologist will then guide you through a set of exercises designed just for you. Personal trainers are good to use if you have no significant problems, but they rarely have formal training in designing programs for people with limitations. And "cookbook" type programs for those who have no specific limitations should be avoided by those with joint problems.

Your physical-fitness program should be set up so that you're gradually doing more intense exercise for longer periods of time, without straining or forcing to the point of injury. The program should include components to improve at least the first four types of fitness (strength, aerobic capacity, flexibility, and agility/balance). While exercising, keep these tips in mind:

- There is a cardinal rule for those who have osteoarthritis: *Never exercise through joint pain!* "No pain, no gain" refers to working through muscle soreness, not joint pain.
- Listen to your body. Stop exercising if you feel dizzy or sick to your stomach, if you're short of breath, or if your chest feels pained or tight.
- Don't overdo it; you may injure yourself. There is a difference between doing a little more in or-

der to improve, and pushing it to the point of injury. Learn to distinguish between the two.

• Keep breathing while you exercise. You may be tempted to hold your breath when you exert yourself, but don't. Your body needs *more* oxygen when you exercise, not less. The blood pressure shoots up when you are straining and holding your breath. (Normal blood pressure is 120/80—Olympic weight lifters have been known to drive their blood pressures all the way up to 480/320!) Holding your breath will also cause lactic acid to accumulate in the muscles, which will increase the amount of muscle soreness you'll feel the next day.

• When you begin your exercise program, you'll probably feel tired, sore, and possibly out of breath. Take it easy, but keep going as long as you can. Eventually your body will adapt. Pretty soon, you'll be surprised at the things that you can do.

• Always cool down after exercising. Don't stop cold after exerting yourself. Instead, stretch, walk, shake out your legs and arms. Stay on your feet, if possible, since sitting down too soon after exercise causes your blood to "pool."

Now let's get into some exercise specifics. Walking, bicycling, and water exercises are the three approaches to fitness many osteoarthritis sufferers find both helpful and enjoyable. (Weight lifting is also critical to treatment but requires a bit more training and has a steeper learning curve.) Let's look at what each has to offer:

WALKING

Walking is perhaps the simplest and easiest aerobic exercise. Like other aerobic activities, walking makes your heart beat faster and your breath come harder. This, in turn, strengthens your cardiovascular system, burns fat, and generally tones and conditions your body. But you've got to do more than stroll at a leisurely pace to get your heart beating faster. You don't have to jog or run, but you do have to keep up a brisk pace. Aerobic walking can be as good for the body as running or bicycling. You burn the same amount of calories by walking as you would running the same distance.

Walking is a low-impact exercise, easy on the joints because they're not jolted by the force of your feet hitting the pavement the way they would be if you were running. (The exception is those who walk at fast paces. At speeds above 5 miles per hour, the impact to the joints is similar, whether walking or jogging.) Walking is inexpensive and requires little equipment other than a comfortable pair of shoes. It's also enjoyable, something you can do with a friend or loved one. Remember to keep the pace up, though, in order to get those all-important aerobic benefits.

To make sure that you're walking fast enough, but not too fast, try the talk-sing test: If you are able to talk while you're walking, without gasping for breath, but haven't enough breath to sing, you're moving at about the right speed. Walking in the "talk-sing" range offers many important benefits, including:

- Increased endurance.
- An overall sense of well-being.
- Greater flexibility in the hips, lower limbs, and possibly the back.
- Improved cardiovascular fitness.
- Greater lung capacity.
- Strengthened muscles in the lower extremities and back.
- Decreased body fat.
- Stronger bones in the lower extremities and hips.
- Improved control of your balance.
- And, in many cases, less osteoarthritis pain.

But before you put your feet to the pavement, remember to:[5]

- Consult your doctor. Ask him or her how long and how vigorously you should walk.
- Wear comfortable shoes, socks to absorb perspiration, and loose, comfortable clothing.
- Spend a few minutes warming up before you begin walking. You can warm up by doing light aerobic exercises to get the blood flowing. Try jumping jacks and "marching in place" (lifting your knees high, one at a time). Simple stretches can also help by loosening muscles, ligaments, and tendons, allowing them to absorb shock bet-

ter while you walk. You can do arm circles and toe touches (but don't bounce or overdo it!).

After you've exercised, spend a few minutes cooling down. Now's the time to stretch for flexibility. (See stretching exercises on pages 136-140.)

- Gradually increase your distance. In the beginning you may want to take a couple of short walks per day rather than one longer walk.
- Walk on flat, solid surfaces—park trails, malls, asphalt or jogging tracks are your best bets for avoiding falls and injuries—until you become a pro.
- For safety's sake, walk during the day, not at night.

Most people with osteoarthritis can walk with little discomfort. But if you have severe hip, knee, ankle, or foot problems, walking may not be the best exercise for you. Ask your doctor or physical therapist to suggest other exercises that may suit you better, like bicycling, for instance.

BICYCLING

Bicycling offers many of the benefits of walking. But since your feet and legs aren't supporting your weight while you pedal, there's less stress and strain on those joints. People with more severe forms of osteoarthritis of the hips, knees, and feet may prefer biking to walking. But remember, bicycling is a limited weight-bearing exercise, so it's not the best approach to building bone strength and density.

Still, bicycling is a great conditioning exercise. It can build up the muscles of the thighs (especially the quadriceps or the front of the thighs) faster than walking. These muscles are the ones that help you get up out of a chair, and they're critical for shock absorption. Moreover, biking is one of the main exercises recommended for those who have knee problems.

Whether you're indoors on a stationary bicycle or outdoors in the fresh air, remember to:[6]

- Warm up for at least five to ten minutes on the bike before tackling any hills (on outdoor bikes) or adding resistance (on stationary bikes).
- Adjust the seat height so that your knees are just slightly bent when the pedal is at its lowest point.
- Make sure you can pedal without too much trouble. Adding resistance should be encouraged as you can handle it. (If using a stationary bike, do not add so much resistance that your pedaling speed drops below 60 revolutions per minute.)
- Pace yourself, especially in the beginning. About 15 to 20 miles per hour should be your initial maximum speed.
- And if you have knee problems you may not want to climb hills on real bicycles, or use resistance on stationary bikes. Get the okay from your doctor first.

WATER EXERCISES

Water exercises are popular with doctors, physical therapists, and patients alike because of the lack of stress and strain on the joints. Sometimes it's the only way that a patient with osteoarthritis can exercise without pain. And three key types of exercise—stretching, strengthening, and aerobic—can easily be done in the water.

You don't have to be an expert swimmer to participate in water exercises, for many of them are done with the help of a flotation device or while standing in the shallow end of the pool. And the benefits of water exercises are numerous, including:[7]

- Decreased pain.
- Support for the body while offering resistance to the muscles as they perform the exercise.
- Easier mobility, which has the added benefit of improved emotional well-being.
- Relaxed muscles.
- Reduced joint compression.
- Social interaction, if you're in a class.
- Improved confidence levels as movement is increased.
- Improved coordination and posture.
- A lower heart rate is maintained, so a higher level of exercise may be tolerated.
- Exercise can sometimes be continued even during a flare-up.

As with any other form of exercise, consult your doctor before you begin a pool program.

Remember that even apparently healthy people should not be alone in the water in case of an emergency. And if you use a colostomy bag or catheter, or have any physical impairments that make it difficult to get in and out of a pool safely, you should look into walking, bicycling, or other exercises instead of swimming.

WEIGHT LIFTING

There are so many specialized weight machines and kinds of free-weight exercises available today, it's almost certain that you'll be able to find at least some that are appropriate for you, no matter what your condition. Some of these machines can be a bit complicated, however, so get some expert instruction in how to use them properly. Weight lifting should not hurt your joints. If it does, you may not be doing the exercise properly, the seat may not be at the right height, or it may just be the wrong exercise for your condition. Get help and advice from an expert, and always listen to your body!

When trying a new exercise, perform the motion with little or no weight until you can do it with the proper form. Then begin to add weight, *but don't worry about how many pounds you are lifting*. The point is to help overcome or prevent osteoarthritis by increasing your muscle strength, not to win an Olympic gold medal. If you can only lift one pound in the beginning, that's fine. Don't strain by trying to lift 100.

You may not want to push yourself to fatigue the first time you do the exercise, for you may be very sore the next day. But as you become familiar with the exercise, increase the amount of weight so that you reach fatigue with about 15 repetitions. Add some more weight and repeat the exercise to fatigue. You will now have done two sets. The first set, with more repetitions, allows you to warm up a bit to prepare for the heavier set. Adjust the number of sets that you do to your muscle-fatigue level. Some days you may need two sets, other days three sets to get the same feeling of fatigue. As long as your joints are not in pain, two sets are better than one, and three are better than two.

When you first start, you may want to limit the number of different exercises you do to about six, making sure that you're working both the upper and lower body. Two sets of six exercises should take only about 20 minutes. As you progress, add new exercises into your routine, and rotate them.

Always remember to exhale during the phase of lifting that has you straining the most. For example, if you're doing the bench press, exhale as you push the weight away from your body, then inhale as you let the weight back down to your chest.

STRETCHING

Stretching is an indispensable part of any good exercise program, but it is especially important to those people with osteoarthritis. If you stretch correctly, you can reap huge benefits. But if you do it incorrectly, you can do an awful lot of damage. Always be careful when stretching, and keep the following guidelines in mind:[8]

- Never stretch a cold muscle; always warm up first. Do your stretching at the *end* of your exercise routine, after you've broken a sweat and have engaged in some aerobic exercise, unless you are playing a sport. Little or no gain in flexibility is made if you stretch first with cold muscles.
- Make sure that you are in the correct position when stretching. It's best to join a class or have an instructor present to make sure that you're not stretching a muscle in the wrong way. Improper stretching can do more damage than good. For most stretches you want to be down on the floor so you can relax your body, especially the area you are stretching. If you don't relax the area you're stretching, your muscles will tighten slightly and you won't make much progress.
- Once you are in the correct position, stretch as far as you can without straining or forcing, then hold your maximum position for 30 seconds. In time, you can increase the hold to 45 seconds.
- Never "bounce" in your stretch, don't keep popping in and out of your maximal stretch. For the best results, relax into the stretch and hold that position. Bouncing can tear muscles, tendons, and ligaments. It also tells the muscles to tighten up just when you want them to relax.

- Don't hold your breath while stretching. Your muscles need the oxygen. Keep breathing, slowly and deeply. Exhale as you try to stretch farther.
- You can triple the effectiveness of your stretching sessions by using PNF (proprioceptive neuromuscular facilitation). Here's how it works: Get into your stretch, as far as you can comfortably go, and hold it. Then contract the muscles in the area you are stretching, without moving the joint. Hold this contraction for 5 to 8 seconds. Then relax the muscle, exhale, and you'll find that you can stretch even farther!
- Stretch at least three times a week, for 20 minutes per session. Stretching two days a week will generally allow you to maintain your current flexibility. Three or more days should bring about improvement.
- Stop if you feel any pain. Pain means you're damaging tissues. You should feel the stretch, but not pain.
- Form is everything. Don't cheat your stretch by contorting your body or using other joints to compensate for inflexibility.
- If you feel any unusual pains or sick in any way, stop and see your physician.

If your joints are quite stiff and you're not used to stretching, you may want to begin by working with a physical therapist, or join a special exercise class for arthritis sufferers. But once you've built up some flexibility, joining a yoga class or the stretch class at your local fitness center may be just the thing to keep you motivated. Feel free to try different classes until you find one that is both challenging and fun, and has an instructor you trust.

There are several good stretches that you can do to loosen up your muscles, tendons, and ligaments and increase your flexibility:

• *For your back and the back of the upper thighs:* Sit on floor with legs apart, arms at your sides. Bend forward and grab your left knee with both hands. If you can bend further, slide your hands down your leg as far as possible. When you have reached your maximum stretch, hold for 30 seconds without bouncing. Slowly bring your upper body to an upright position. Then repeat with your right knee. Spread your legs farther apart and repeat the exercise.

• *For shoulders:* Stand or sit erect. Lift your right arm straight up, then bend it down and behind your head until your right hand touches your upper back (at the opposite shoulder blade, if possible). Reach your left hand over your head, grab your right elbow, and gently pull your right elbow toward your left shoulder. You should feel a good stretch in your right shoulder and upper arm. Hold for 15 seconds. Release. Repeat with other arm.

• *For lower back and hips:* Lie on your back on the floor. Bend your right knee and bring it up toward your chest. Place both hands behind your knee and gently pull it toward your chest. Hold at your maximum stretch for 15 seconds. Repeat with other knee.

• *For calves:* Stand a foot or two away from a wall or sturdy piece of furniture. Keeping your body straight (don't bend at the waist), lean forward, and brace yourself against the wall or furniture. Keep both heels on the ground (very important!). Slowly press both hips forward until you feel the stretch in your calves. If you don't feel the stretch, stand further away from the wall or furniture and try again.

• *Fronts of thighs:* Lie facedown on a mat or carpeted surface. Bend your right knee, grabbing your foot with your left hand. Hold for 30 seconds. Repeat with the other leg.

These are just a few of the countless stretches you can do. Ask your doctor or physical therapist for more.

Getting Started

"I love the *idea* of exercise," a veteran couch potato once said, quite seriously. "It's actually *doing* it that I can't stand."

That's a common complaint. We all understand why exercise is good but find it hard to get started. Well, the key is simply to *get started*. And to help you do this, let's sweep aside the common arguments against exercise.

• *I haven't exercised for so long, I won't be able to do it.* Don't worry about it. Your doctor and your physical therapist will develop a special exercise program that's geared to your capabilities.

• *Exercise hurts.* You may be a little sore or stiff in the beginning, as your body adapts to the new movements and demands. But exercise, properly done, should not be painful. Pain means that you're either overdoing it or doing it incorrectly. Tell your doctor or therapist about any discomfort or continuous pain.

• *It takes too long to see results.* Ask your doctor or physical therapist to design a program that allows you to meet small goals quickly and consistently. A little success can make you a convert.

• *There isn't enough time to exercise.* If you haven't time for a half hour of walking or bicycling, followed by a warm-down and stretching session, remember that several short exercise periods can be just as effective as one longer period. So take advantage of lulls during the day to squeeze in a little exercise. Ask your doctor for exercises you can do while you're at work, standing in the bank line, or sitting in your car in a traffic jam. Seize any brief moment to loosen your joints and get fit.

• *Exercising is boring.* Some exercises *will* bore you. So will some foods, movies, and books. The trick is to find one or more types of exercise that you enjoy. If you love the outdoors, walking or bicycling are excellent choices. If you love the feeling of being in water, swimming or water exercises may be for you. If you prefer to be indoors, yoga or dancing may be just right. Try exercising with a friend or family member. Join an exercise class. Listen to your favorite music during exercise. Walk through a park instead of around your neighborhood. Whatever exercise you do, make it as pleasant and enjoyable as possible. There's an exercise just right for you. If you look, you'll find it.

Quick Tips to Improve Exercise Motivation and Compliance

- *Get a workout partner.* If someone is waiting for you on the corner at 5:30 A.M., you'll be more likely to get up and out instead of sleeping in and skipping your workout.
- *Keep an exercise log.* This can be as simple as placing a red X on a calendar on the days you exercise, or it may be as complex as jotting down the specifics about your workout in a notebook.
- *Get new clothes/shoes/toys.* Without busting your budget, buy the fancy bicycle shorts or aerobics leotard you've always admired. Devices, such as a heart-rate monitor, can also be very motivating.
- *Train for a competition or an event.* If you've got a goal, you'll work harder.
- *Do cross training or seasonal training.* This helps prevent boredom and works different parts of the body in different ways. Always make sure you've got an indoor activity to do in case of bad weather.
- *Keep equipment in plain sight.* Don't hide your tennis racquet in a distant closet. Keep it out, where you can see it as a reminder to get moving!

- *Work out in the morning.* If you work out first thing in the morning you'll have gotten your exercise in, no matter how busy your day becomes.
- *Combine your workout with work.* Many people walk or bike to work or find ways to do some exercise during their lunch hour.
- *Ease up on days when you're not feeling strong.* You don't always drive a car in fifth gear; sometimes you have to downshift. On your "down" days, doing just a few minutes of exercise is far better than skipping it completely.
- *Subscribe to a magazine.* For about $1.50 a month, you get a reminder to exercise.
- *Try the 5-Minute Rule.* On days when you just don't feel motivated, plan on exercising for just 5 minutes. If you still don't feel like exercising after 5 minutes, quit. Most of the time, though, you'll start feeling invigorated and you'll continue.

Get Started!

Some people are reluctant to exercise because they fear they'll "wear out" their joints or damage them further if they already have osteoarthritis. Their fears sound reasonable but are not supported by facts. Most scientists and doctors believe that even vigorous exercise *does not* cause osteoarthritis to develop in normal joints. In fact, it's just the opposite. The flowing of synovial fluid into and out of the cartilage *counteracts* damage in normal joints.

Exercises that involve high stress-repetitive

movements, such as pitching a baseball hundreds of thousands of times, can trigger *secondary osteoarthritis*. And those who engage in sports at highly competitive levels with injured joints are also at an increased risk for developing osteoarthritis. The bottom line is this: Use common sense when exercising. Avoid specific exercises or activities that place abnormal stress on your joints. But *do* find some kind of activity that feels comfortable and start moving! Although glucosamine and chondroitin sulfates will help rebuild damaged cartilage, you need to exercise regularly in order to ensure good joint health.

7

◇

Healthy Eating Really Counts

How can I reduce my osteoarthritis symptoms by changing my diet?

What foods can cause or reduce inflammation?

How can fish oils help ease osteoarthritis symptoms?

What can evening primrose oil do for osteoarthritis?

What role do bioflavonoids play in an osteoarthritis diet?

What is the "antioxidant connection"?

What are the best ways to maintain or reduce my weight?

What effect do aspirin and other pain medications have on my nutritional status?

Do other "arthritis diets" help?

You've heard all the clichés: "You are what you eat." "Food is the best medicine." "Your body is like a car and it needs the best fuel in order to run properly." Like most clichés, these are based on fact. What we choose to put into our bodies can either strengthen or weaken us, making us more or less healthy while increasing or decreasing the symptoms of disease. This chapter tells you how to fuel your body with health-enhancing foods, some of which can lessen and may even help prevent some of the symptoms of osteoarthritis. If you follow these dietary guidelines, you'll also be beefing up your immune system and lowering your chances of getting heart disease, cancer, stroke, and diabetes—some of America's biggest killer diseases. We'll also discuss the essentials of a good diet, foods that may help to hinder osteoarthritis, the use of antioxidants and other supplements, the effects of certain medications on nutrient needs, and the key essentials of weight control.

What Makes Up a Healthy Diet?

It's relatively easy to eat well enough to prevent a major vitamin or mineral deficiency disease such as beriberi or scurvy. But a minor deficiency of any nutrient can leave the body in a weakened state, more susceptible to disease and less equipped to fight off invaders.

Your body needs many different nutrients to keep running in peak form, including protein, carbohydrates, fats, fiber, vitamins, minerals, and phytochemicals. These are found in different combinations and different amounts in various foods. If you continually eat the same foods over and over (even foods high in nutrients), you may be missing out on important building blocks for your health. Not only is variety the spice of life, it's the spark-plug of health.

Stopping the Joint Busters

Researchers have consistently found that consuming a healthful diet is one of the most important things we can do to safeguard our health. But exciting news for osteoarthritis sufferers is emerging from scientific labs concerning a special connection between food and the symptoms of osteoarthritis. Certain foods can help stem the destruction of joints, while others may help to ease the pain or prevent the problem in the first place.

Several theories attempt to explain why our joints deteriorate. One of the most widely accepted holds that certain unstable molecules called *free radicals* roam about the body attacking and destroying healthy tissue, including the tissue found in the joints.

Free radicals are unstable because they have lost or gained electrons, making them erratic and very reactive with their environment. In an effort to stabilize themselves, free radical molecules "steal" electrons from other molecules, disrupting their victims' structures and damaging whatever tissues those molecules are part of.[1] Free radicals are thought to be a major cause of many diseases, including cancer, heart disease, and aging and degenerative diseases. Osteoarthritis may be the result of free radical damage. And, to make matters worse, joint inflammation itself may trigger an even faster rate of new free radical formation. Prevention of free radical damage is a critical feature in treating and preventing osteoarthritis.

Luckily, help in fighting free radicals is available in the form of the *antioxidants*. The antioxidants are so-named because they serve as antidotes to one of the free radicals most commonly found in the body—oxygen. No, it's not regular oxygen that we all need to breathe to stay alive. This is a special, unstable form of oxygen called *singlet oxygen*. Oxygen molecules usually travel in groups of two. But sometimes, during the normal metabolic processes in the body, twosomes split, forming two separate molecules of singlet oxygen. Singlet oxygen is highly reactive and causes a great deal of damage as it struggles to stabilize itself by stealing electrons from other molecules. The antioxidants "quench" singlet oxygen, stabilizing it and preventing it from attacking bodily tissues.[2]

Where can you find antioxidants? They're as close as your refrigerator or your nearest bottle of vitamins. The antioxidants include vitamin A (or beta carotene and other carotenoids, which are the plant form of the vitamin), vitamin C, vitamin E, and the mineral selenium. An easy way to remember them is A, C, E, and the S in selenium spell the word "ACES." Foods that contain any of the four ACES are powerful weapons for combating free radicals and the havoc that they wreak. It's best to get your ACES from whole foods, rather than from supplements, for when they're in the foods the antioxidants are mixed in with other substances that can be critical in disease prevention. Here are some good food sources of the ACES:

• *Vitamin A, beta carotene, the carotenoids.* Researchers have discovered that the carotenoids (beta carotene, the plant form of vitamin A, is one of dozens) are very effective in fighting free radicals. Carotenoids are found mostly in yellow-orange fruits and vegetables such as apricots, sweet potatoes, pumpkin, carrots, cantaloupe and other melons, mangoes, papaya, peaches, and winter squash, as well as the dark green leafy vegetables such as broccoli, spinach, collard greens, parsley, and other leafy greens.[3] If you cut open a fruit or vegetable and see color inside, chances are that it is a good source of carotenoids. You'll find vitamin

A in liver, turkey, milk, and other foods of animal origin.

• *Vitamin C.* This antioxidant is found in many delicious fresh fruits such as cantaloupe, grapefruit, papaya, kiwi, oranges, mangoes, raspberries, pineapples, bananas, strawberries, and tomatoes and fresh vegetables such as Brussels sprouts, collard greens, cabbage, asparagus, broccoli, potatoes, and red peppers.[4] Fruits and vegetables should be as fresh as possible and, if cooked, should be steamed or microwaved only a short time, for vitamin C is heat sensitive and easily destroyed by cooking or processing. Cutting these foods after cooking them (rather than before) helps to maintain vitamin C content.

• *Vitamin E.* The primary sources of this antioxidant are vegetable oils (such as sunflower and safflower), sunflower seeds, wheat germ, nuts, avocados, peaches, whole-grain breads and cereals, spinach, broccoli, asparagus, dried prunes, and peanut butter.[5]

• *Selenium:* Besides protecting the cells from the toxic effects of free radicals, some evidence suggests that selenium can help to keep the immune system functioning properly. You can find good amounts of selenium in swordfish, salmon, tuna, cracked wheat bread, sunflower seeds, oysters, and shrimp.[6]

Again, it's always best to get the vitamins and minerals that your body needs from fresh, whole foods rather than from supplements. Unfortunately, the content of many of the antioxidants and minerals in food can vary quite a bit. For example, one stalk of broccoli may have ten times more selenium than another stalk, because the soil in which it was grown was a richer source of the mineral. That's why it will probably be necessary to take supplements in order to help treat and prevent osteoarthritis. The generally recommended dosages for antioxidant supplements are:

- Vitamin A—5,000 IU
- Vitamin C—500 to 4,000 mg
- Vitamin E—100 to 400 IU
- Selenium—55 to 200 mcg

Strengthening the Joints with Bioflavonoids

The bioflavonoids, a group of substances found in virtually all plant foods, are essential for healthy capillary walls and the metabolism of vitamin C.[8] There are more than 4,000 different types of bioflavonoids. Some of them help osteoarthritis sufferers by:

- Reinforcing the ability of collagen to form a strong matrix.
- Preventing free radical damage.
- Slowing the inflammation response.
- Preventing collagen from being destroyed when the cartilage tissue is inflamed.
- Hastening the healing of athletic injury.

———————◇———————

Boron—This mineral is not considered a true antioxidant but does possess some antioxidant function. It is important in maintaining joint health and helps to keep some cells from releasing free radicals. In geographic areas where boron intakes are low, osteoarthritis incidence is high and vice versa. Also, some studies have shown that boron can have a beneficial effect on osteoarthritis.[7] Cauliflower and apples with their skins are good sources of boron. For supplementation, the recommended dosage is 3 mg for adults.

———————◇———————

The foods with the greatest concentrations of bioflavonoids include green tea, berries, onions, citrus fruits, and fruits that contain a pit (such as cherries and plums). Other sources include fresh fruits, fresh vegetables, seeds, and whole grains. Bioflavonoids are sold in supermarkets and health food stores as citrus bioflavonoids, rutin, quercetin, hesperidin, catechins, gingko biloba extracts, milk thistle seed extracts, and wine proanthocyanidins. They are usually included in multivitamins or minerals, vitamin C, and antioxidant supplements.[9]

Bad Medicine for Your Nutrient Status

Despite their best efforts, many people find themselves suffering from nutrient deficiencies caused

————————◇————————

Foods contain varying amounts of antioxidants, and some people absorb them better than do others, so it's difficult to tell if you are getting all that you need. That's why a test of your antioxidant function is often helpful. This specialized test (performed by SpectraCell Labs in Houston, among others) doesn't just measure the amounts of antioxidants in your body. Instead, it looks at how well your antioxidant systems are functioning. The results are given as a percentile ranking, along with recommendations for repletion.

If you have a less-than-ideal antioxidant function percentile, but seem to be taking the recommended doses of the main antioxidant supplements, you may want to look into other antioxidants such as proanthocyanidins (pycnogenol, 30-100 mg), curcumin (100–500 mg), garlic (100–500 mg), cysteine (n-acetyl-l-cysteine, 250–1,000 mg), coenzyme Q10 (10–100 mg), and bioflavonoids.

————————◇————————

by common prescription and over-the-counter medicines. Taking medications, especially on a long-term basis, can affect the way your body absorbs and retains key nutrients.[10] You may be surprised to learn, for example, that taking high doses of simple *aspirin* (12 or more per day) can cause your body to absorb less vitamin C while excreting greater amounts, lose iron through gastrointestinal bleeding, and decrease the folic acid levels in the blood.[11] And indomethacin, also know by its trade name, Indocin, is an NSAID that can cause water retention and iron loss, and decrease levels of vitamin C in the blood. To combat these problems, be sure to eat foods high in vitamin C, iron, and also folic acid if taking aspirin. You'll find vitamin C in red peppers and citrus fruits, folic acid in dark green leafy vegetables, and iron in organ meats such as liver and heart and whole-grain breads and cereals. If your iron loss is significant, you may wish to take supplements, but be aware that *excess iron* can be a problem in some people (especially middle-aged men). Before supplementing with iron, consider checking with your physician and getting a blood test called ferritin, which checks your iron levels. Excess iron levels could indicate a metabolic condition called hemochromatosis, which can cause secondary osteoarthritis among other serious conditions. This condition is not rare, yet it is not routinely screened for on the blood tests you have with a yearly physical exam.

Antacids containing aluminum or magnesium hydroxide are often taken to counteract the gastrointestinal problems that accompany the use of NSAIDs. But over time these antacids can lower the amount of phosphorus that your body absorbs.[13] You may need to counter the loss of this vital mineral by eating phosphorus-rich foods including lean meat, fish, lean poultry, nonfat milk or yogurt, cooked soybeans, peanut butter, whole-wheat breads, cooked broccoli, oranges, bananas, cooked carrots, nuts, and seeds.

Corticosteroids are prescribed when there is severe joint pain or inflammation and other painkillers just haven't worked. In addition to a host of side effects, corticosteroids can wreak havoc on your nutrient status. They can cause water retention, decreased absorption of vitamin D, and a faster rate of excretion of zinc, potassium, and vitamin C, which can lead to deficiencies.[14] Since steroids are only prescribed in extreme circumstances, your doctor will undoubtedly monitor your body's reaction to these very powerful drugs. However, you may want to decrease your sodium (salt) intake and eat more of the following foods to compensate for the faster excretion and decreased absorption:

- *Zinc:* oysters, whole-grain breads and cereals, brewer's yeast
- *Potassium:* bananas, orange juice, dried fruits
- *Vitamin C:* citrus fruits, red peppers, potatoes

Medicines are sometimes necessary but are often a threat to healthy nutrient status. Be sure to ask your physician if the medicines you are taking interfere with your absorption or utilization of any nutrients and, if so, what to do. Once you start taking the Arthritis Cure, though, the need for these nutrient-robbing medicines disappears.

Controlling Inflammation

Inflammation can be the source of much pain and discomfort for the owner of an osteoarthritic joint, occuring most often in the more advanced cases. Inflammation is the body's natural response to tissue damage, or to overuse of a diseased joint. Although well-intentioned, the inflammation response is what may make your joints feel stiff, warm, swollen, and achy.

Inflammation is one of the ways the body protects itself after injury or disease. When tissue is damaged, the white blood cells race to the "scene of the crime." There they produce substances called *prostaglandins* and *leukotrienes*, which bring on a multitude of biochemical reactions including inflammation. Fatty acids can alter this inflammation response, either for the better or for the worse. For instance, *arachidonic acid* (which is found in animal products) can increase inflammation, while *alpha-linolenic acid (ALA), eicosapentaenoic acid (EPA), gamma-linolenic acid (GLA)*, and *linoleic acid* can all reduce it. If inflammation is a problem for you, be aware that you can either increase or decrease the swelling and pain in your joints by eating certain foods.[15]

The Inflammation Fighters

Let's first take a look at the fatty acids that can reduce inflammation:[16]

———————◇———————

In addition to the prostaglandins and leukotrienes, the white blood cells produce free radicals and hydrogen peroxide, which help to damage the cartilage.

———————◇———————

Alpha-linolenic acid (ALA) is found in green vegetables and other foods of plant origin. ALA is an omega-3 fatty acid, the kind that blocks the production of those overzealous prostaglandins and leukotrienes.

Gamma-linolenic acid (GLA), found in black currant oil, evening primrose oil, and borage seed oil, is a precursor of the "good" prostaglandins. That's right—not all prostaglandins are bad. Some prostaglandins prevent blood platelets from sticking together, improve the blood flow, and *reduce* inflammation. GLA helps to make these "good" prostaglandins. (Unfortunately, these oils have also been shown to *trigger* inflammation in some people, so be cautious if you decide to take them.)

Linoleic acid is found in plant oils such as corn, soybean, sunflower, safflower, flaxseed, and other light vegetable oils. Linoleic acid helps the body increase its level of EPA, which in turn blocks the production of harmful prostaglandins.

Eicosapentaenoic acid (EPA), the best known of the omega-3 fatty acids, is found in marine plants and fish. EPA is actually made by algae, plankton, and seaweed, which are then eaten by certain fish. Not all fish are good sources of EPAs—much of the white fish found in the United States doesn't have much. Coldwater fatty fish caught in the ocean have the greatest amounts, including mackerel, anchovies, herring, salmon, sardines, lake trout, Atlantic sturgeon, and tuna. Eating as little as one ounce of fish per day or two fish meals per week can help reduce inflammation. (Be aware that deep-frying destroys omega-3 fatty acids, besides adding loads of unhealthful fat.)

Although it's always better to get your nutrients from real food, some people take their omega-3s in supplement form (fish oil capsules). Be careful not to overdo either method of consumption, however, since too much fish or fish oil can interfere with your blood's ability to clot. And excessive intake of fish oil can lead to overdoses of vitamins A and D (especially if you're getting A and D in your vitamin supplements), which can be toxic.

The Inflammation Producer

Arachidonic acid is the main food culprit when it comes to producing inflammation. Originating almost entirely in animal products and saturated fats, it is a precursor to the "bad" kind of prostaglandins that produce platelet stickiness, hardening of the arteries, heart disease, and strokes, as well as inflammation. Meat, poultry, dairy products (especially those containing saturated fat), and egg yolks all contain arachidonic acid.

Maintaining or Losing Weight— What You Need to Know

Excess weight can cause secondary osteoarthritis, specifically of the knees. The problem may be due to the extra weight alone or perhaps to an obesity-related metabolic change. But by reducing your weight (if you're overweight), you can either prevent the development of osteoarthritis of the weight-bearing joints or dramatically reduce its symptoms.

Following stringent diets, especially those that are based upon just a few foods, doesn't work for long-term weight loss. You may lose weight initially, but once the "diet" is ended, the pounds pile on in a hurry, and you may end up with more body fat than before you started. People who fall into the "yo-yo" trap of dieting, losing then gaining over and over again, become fatter and have a higher mortality rate than those who remain at a constant weight, even if that weight is high. In the long run, it's what you do on a daily basis that makes the difference. That's why it's important to adopt a sensible, flexible, and easy-to-follow eating plan.

How do you get control of your weight? Most people who have successfully lost weight and kept

————————◇————————

The Japanese government has an interesting approach to dietary recommendations. They suggest eating at least 30 different foods a day. By eating many different kinds of foods, it's almost certain that you will get a wide variety of nutrients—unless it's 30 different kinds of junk food! And most people can't "overdose" on any one kind of food when they have 29 other kinds to fit into their diets.

————————◇————————

it off have certain characteristics in common. They include:

• *Making changes for themselves, not to please others.* Internal motivation is the key. You have to want to lose weight, keep fit, and reduce your osteoarthritis symptoms. You can't do it just because your spouse or your best friend has nagged you into it.

• *Focusing on fitness.* Rather than looking at numbers on a scale to see how well you're doing, focus on how much farther you can walk each day, or how many more repetitions of an exercise you can do than you did when you started. A formerly obese person who can now run a seven-minute mile rarely continues to have an obesity problem.

• *Doing at least some exercise each day.* Keeping your body in motion raises your basic metabolic rate and burns calories faster than before—even when resting! The more you exercise, the more calories you can take in while still losing weight.

• *Never skipping meals*. Skipping meals (especially breakfast) can slow your basal metabolic rate. Also, when you skip meals or go too long without eating, it's hard not to overeat at the next meal and not to choose fatty, sugary foods.

• *Watching the fat intake*. Fat is a concentrated source of calories, so it's easy to hike up your caloric intake by eating just a small amount. It's important to get *some* fat each day (the equivalent of about 1 tablespoon), but most people consume much more than this. Limiting fat intake is probably the easiest and most efficient way of lowering caloric intake.

• *Using alcohol in small quantities, if at all*. Alcohol provides very little nutrition, but (depending upon what it's mixed with and how much you drink) it can add a whopping number of calories to your diet. Alcohol also lowers inhibitions, possibly encouraging excess eating. In fact, a significant portion of the obese population might be slimmer if they drank less. It's best and safest to avoid alcohol completely, but if you drink, do so in moderation.

• *Never counting calories or "dieting."* People who are successful at losing and maintaining their weight do not follow stringent "diets" or burden themselves with calorie counting. Strict diets and calorie counts are too restrictive and burdensome, quickly dropped in favor of a more "tolerable" way of living. It's a much better idea to adopt a flexible, easy-to-follow general food plan that includes all the kinds of foods that you need to maintain health while slimming.

• *Not weighing themselves more than once a week.* It's normal for body weight to fluctuate a few pounds during the course of a single day, mostly due to changes in water content. Those who weigh themselves daily (or worse yet, several times a day) may become obsessed with the numbers on the scale, panicked when there is a slight gain, or overly confident when there is a loss. Their eating becomes dictated by the scale.

• *Being content with their bodies and realistic about their goals.* If you are 5-foot-9 and 325 pounds, don't obsess over the idea that you should weigh 125 pounds, and if you don't you're a failure. Accept yourself as you are today, while working to improve (even just a little bit) every day from now on.

• *Being organized.* Successful weight managers prepare in advance for events by eating full, well-balanced meals at home and, if necessary, bringing their own food along. They are committed to their goals. They arrange their schedules so that they always have time for meals and their exercise sessions, the most important meeting of the day.

• *Understanding the reasons for their overeating and past failures.* People eat for many reasons besides physical hunger. Many use food to quell pain or ease boredom, or just because they like the oral stimulation. Once you figure out why you overeat, substitute another activity. For instance, during my frequent breaks at work I used to slip something in my mouth to give myself a time-out. Then I realized I wasn't really hungry, so I decided to substitute a healthier behavior. I now throw darts at my dart board or visit with a colleague down the hall during my break time.

Putting It All Together: Eating to Beat Osteoarthritis

We've covered a lot of nutritional ground. Now it's time to put it all together. The five elements of a powerful anti-osteoarthritis diet are foods filled with antioxidants, foods that contain bioflavonoids, foods that counter the ill effects of medications, foods that reduce inflammation, and foods that enable you to keep your weight under control. Let's see exactly what you can eat to incorporate into your diet these five ways to fight osteoarthritis.

OSTEOARTHRITIS FIGHTER 1 *Foods That Contain Antioxidants*

Vitamin A/carotenoids. Yellow-orange fruits and vegetables such as apricots, sweet potatoes, pumpkin, carrots, cantaloupe, mangoes, papaya, peaches, and winter squash. Also dark green leafy vegetables such as broccoli, spinach, collard greens, parsley, and other leafy greens.

Vitamin C. Cantaloupe, grapefruit, papaya, kiwi, oranges, mangoes, raspberries, pineapples, bananas, strawberries, tomatoes, Brussels sprouts, collard greens, cabbage, asparagus, broccoli, potatoes, and red peppers.

Vitamin E. Vegetable oils (sunflower and safflower), sunflower seeds, wheat germ, nuts, avocados, peaches, whole-grain breads and cereals, spinach, broccoli, asparagus, dried prunes, and peanut butter.

Selenium. Swordfish, salmon, tuna, cracked wheat bread, selenium-rich yeast, sunflower seeds, oysters, and shrimp.

Summing Up #1: To Get Plenty of Antioxidants . . .

Eat at least one food from the vitamin A/carotenoids list and two from the vitamin C list daily. One tablespoon oil or one other food from the vitamin E list daily is sufficient, and one selenium-rich food per week.

If you wish to take supplements, check with your doctor. Nutritionally minded physicians generally consider these to be safe ranges for most adults: vitamin A (5,000 IU); vitamin C (500–1,000 mg); vitamin E (100–400 IU), selenium (55–200 mcg), boron (3 mg).

OSTEOARTHRITIS FIGHTER _____ 2 *Foods That Contain Bioflavonoids*

You'll find bioflavonoids in citrus fruits, berries, green tea, onions, fruits that contain a pit (such as cherries and plums), and whole grains. Eat at least one food rich in bioflavonoids per day. If you wish to supplement, most nutritionists agree that you should take 100 milligrams bioflavonoids for every 500 milligrams of vitamin C.

OSTEOARTHRITIS FIGHTER _____ 3 *Foods That Counter the Use of NSAIDs, Steroids, and Other Medications*

Vitamin C. See the list above.

Iron. Organ meats (liver, heart, kidney, etc.), lean red meat, cooked dried beans and peas, dark leafy vegetables, fish, poultry, prunes and prune juice, oysters, whole-grain breads, and cereals.

Folic Acid. Brewer's yeast, dark green leafy vegetables, orange juice, liver, avocados, beets, and broccoli.

Phosphorus. Meat, organ meats, fish, poultry, eggs, nonfat milk, low-fat yogurt, soybeans, and peanut butter.

Zinc. Oysters, lean meat, poultry, fish, organ meats, whole-grain breads and cereals, brewer's yeast, and pumpkin seeds.

Potassium. Lean meats, potatoes, avocados, bananas, apricots, orange juice, dried fruits, cooked dried beans, and peas.

Summing Up #3: To Counteract the Nutritionally Harmful Effects of Medicines ...

Aspirin takers: Eat an extra serving of foods high in vitamin C, iron, and folic acid each day.

Indomethacin takers: Eat an iron-rich food each day and watch sodium/salt intake.

Antacid takers: Eat a phosphorus-rich food each day.

Corticosteroid takers: Eat an extra serving of foods containing zinc, potassium, and vitamin C each day. Drink vitamin D–enriched milk. Concentrate on low-fat, low-calorie foods to counteract increased appetite.

OSTEOARTHRITIS
FIGHTER _____ 4 *Foods that Reduce Inflammation*

Omega-3 fatty acids—The most effective type of omega-3 fatty acids are the EPAs, which are found in coldwater fish that are caught in the wild. Omega-3s are the best natural inflammation fighters, and EPA is the best of the omega-3s. Mackerel, anchovies, herring, salmon, sardines, lake trout, Atlantic sturgeon, and tuna are good sources of EPA. (But don't deep-fry.) Eating 2 to 5 fish meals per week is recommended. If you don't eat fish you may want to take 1 to 2 teaspoons of fish oil per day. (*NOTE: Do not take more than the recommended dose of fish oil, as fish oil can be toxic in large amounts and can interfere with blood clotting. See your doctor before taking any fish oil.*)

Evening primrose oil, black currant oil, and borage seed oil—These oils all contain gamma-linolenic acid (GLA), which is an acceptable (although less effective) substitute for EPA. However, GLA may, in rare cases, trigger inflammation in some people, so use with caution. These oils will work with your diet, but they do tend to be expensive. A standard dose is 200 to 300 milligrams (they come in capsule form), but check with your doctor.

Plant oils such as corn, soybean, sunflower, safflower, or flaxseed—These contain linoleic acid, which helps the body increase EPA levels and thus lessens the inflammatory response. One tablespoon per day should be helpful for most people.

Summing Up #4: To Use Your Diet to Help Lessen the Inflammation Response, Either ...

- Eat 2 to 5 fish meals per week; *or* take 1 to 2 teaspoons fish oil daily; *or*
- Take 200 to 300 milligrams of evening primrose oil, black current oil, or borage seed oil; *or*
- Take 1 tablespoon of the plant oils listed above.

OSTEOARTHRITIS
FIGHTER _____ 5 *Keeping Your Weight Under Control*

Follow the Food Guide Pyramid when selecting foods and amounts for your basic eating plan. Take supplements as indicated. Concentrate on lower fat, nutrient-rich foods. Do not skip meals or "diet" to lose weight. Put most of your time and energy into fitness, especially improving your aerobic capacity and strength. And remember to make changes gradually, sticking with them until they become second nature.

Arthritis Diet Myths

A good diet can help you control some of the symptoms of osteoarthritis. But there is no single diet that can "cure" arthritis. Beware of diets that require an excessive amount of one food or nutrient, or diets that require you to leave out entire food groups. And watch out for these three popular dietary myths:

• **Diet Myth #1:** *Removing "nightshade" vegetables from your diet can relieve sore joints.* This myth emerged in the 1960s when a horticulturist from Rutgers University noticed that he personally experienced sore joints after eating "nightshade" vegetables. Nightshades come from the plant genus *Solanum* and include more than 1,700 herbs, shrubs, and trees, including eggplant, bell peppers, potatoes, and tomatoes.[17] Although there are many claims that removing nightshades will cure arthritis, no scientific proof has been offered.

• **Diet Myth #2:** *The Dong Diet can significantly improve the symptoms of arthritis.* The Dong Diet is an elimination diet developed by Collin Dong, M.D., patterned after the diet that many Chinese have followed for centuries. The diet calls for the elimination of all preservatives, additives, fruits, red meat, herbs, alcohol, and dairy products. There is absolutely no scientific proof that this diet works.

• **Diet Myth #3:** *A "natural" diet rich in alfalfa can reduce the symptoms of arthritis.* Alfalfa taken in high doses can actually interfere with normal blood cell production. And a good diet needs to include a great deal more than just high amounts of a certain food.

Fad diets for osteoarthritis will come and go, but the safe and sound principles remain the same.

A Therapeutic Diet for Osteoarthritis Sufferers

Here is a full day's worth of sample menus to help you get started. Be creative, use many different kinds of fruits, vegetables, and whole grains rather than eating the same few over and over again. Try fruits and vegetables you've never had before. This is meant only as a guide. Be sure to discuss any changes in your diet with your physician.

If you are trying to lose weight, eat the lesser number of recommended servings and omit the optional servings. (Serving sizes are detailed below.)

BREAKFAST
2 to 3 servings bread/cereal (whole grains preferred)
1 serving milk or yogurt (nonfat preferred)
1 serving fruit

LUNCH
2 to 3 servings bread/cereal (whole grains preferred)
1 serving fish, lean poultry, or meat (occasionally), or cooked dried beans or peas
1 to 2 servings vegetables
1 to 2 servings fruit
1 serving milk or yogurt (nonfat preferred)

SNACK
1 bread (optional)
1 fruit (optional)

DINNER
   2 to 3 servings bread/cereal (whole grains pre-
         ferred)
   1 to 2 servings fish, lean poultry, or meat (occa-
         sionally), or cooked dried beans or peas
   2 to 3 servings vegetables
   1 serving fruit (optional)

SNACK
   1 serving bread (optional)
   1 serving milk or yogurt (nonfat preferred)

Avoid heavily marbled or fatty meats, the dark
meat or skin of poultry, visible fat, and egg yolk since
they contain the inflammation-inducing arachidonic
acid. You may wish to supplement your diet with
omega-3 fatty acids, antioxidants, minerals, and/or
bioflavonoids. If so, consult with your doctor.

   Following are some suggestions for serving sizes
from each of the food groups. Although there's no
such thing as a "one size fits all" eating plan, these
are general guidelines everyone can follow.

Bread, cereal, rice, and pasta (6–11 servings)—This
group should make up the largest portion of your
diet, providing much-needed carbohydrates, fiber,
energy, B vitamins, and sometimes iron. A typical
serving from this group would be one piece of
bread, ½ to 1 cup of cereal, or ½ cup of cooked rice
or pasta. In general, whole-grain products are more
nutritious than refined products.

Vegetables (3–5 servings)—The vegetable group provides important vitamins such as vitamin C and folic acid, minerals, fiber, the carotenoids and plant substances called phytochemicals. A serving of vegetables is made up of 1 cup of raw vegetables, ½ cup cooked vegetables, or ¾ cup vegetable juice. (Juice should only be counted as one serving per day, for it lacks much-needed fiber.)

Fruit (2–4 servings)—Vitamin C, carotenoids, and fiber are among the contributions of the fruit group. One medium fruit, ½ cup juice, or 1 cup chopped fruit constitutes a serving. Once again, only ½ cup of juice should be counted toward your fruit allotment per day.

Meat, poultry, fish, dried beans, and eggs (2–3 servings)—A serving of this group (which provides protein, riboflavin, and vitamins B_6, B_{12}, and others) may be smaller than you'd expect—just 2 to 3 ounces of cooked, lean meat, poultry, or fish, or ½ cup of cooked dried beans, or one egg. We used to believe that we needed lots of protein to stay healthy, but we now know that most Americans are "over proteinized." Remember that trimming the fat, removing the skin, and choosing the leaner cuts of meat and poultry can make the difference between a high-fat, high-calorie choice and a "slimmer" one. Try to limit your intake of beef. When you do choose it, remember that a cut with the word "round" in its name, such as "round steak," is generally lower in fat. Fish, as we'll explain later, is an excellent choice, especially since its omega-3 fatty acids have been linked to heart health and a lowered inflammation response.

Milk, yogurt, and cheese (2–3 servings)—This group provides calcium, vitamin D, protein, and other nutrients important for growth and maintenance of strong bones and connective tissues. One serving equals one cup of milk, 1½ ounces of natural cheese, 2 ounces of processed cheese, or 1 cup of yogurt. Remember that most cheeses are high in fat and calories, so opt for nonfat and low-fat choices whenever possible. Nonfat milk and yogurt are also better choices than their richer counterparts, while providing the same beneficial nutrients.

8

◇

Beating the Blues

What is depression?

What is the link between depression and osteoarthritis?

What are the signs of depression?

Who is at risk for becoming depressed?

How can I beat the blues?

What are antidepressants?

What are "keeping up" and "covering up"?

How do stress and fatigue worsen depression?

How can I make my body more stress and fatigue resistant?

How can I get a better night's sleep?

Robin's problem began very slowly. At first she simply slept a little later every morning and felt slightly fatigued when she woke up. But two years after it began, she was tired all the time. Routine chores exhausted her, and she had no energy for her husband or her friends. Thinking that it might be a problem with her endocrine system, her immune system, her nervous system, or her heart, a phalanx of doctors put her through a variety of tests and wound up prescribing "a bunch of medicines, I forgot how many." Of course the drugs had side effects, including depression, so new drugs had to be used to quell the harmful effects of the old ones. The doctors never found anything to explain Robin's fatigue. The only thing wrong with this otherwise textbook-healthy 35-year-old woman was rather severe osteoarthritis of the right knee.

Osteoarthritis: That was the problem. Not directly, for osteoarthritis does not cause fatigue or emotional upset. But anything that produces pain, limits mobility, and threatens disability can lead to depression, which, in turn, can result in fatigue, listlessness, lack of interest in family and friends, sexual difficulties, and many other problems. It turns out that Robin had been a very promising fencer, possibly a candidate for the Olympics, when at age 23 osteoarthritis of her right knee, her "lunging knee," forced her to set aside her sword. All at once, her dreams were shattered and her future ripped away. She became depressed. And her unhappiness deepened as the pain in her knee grew, forcing her to give up the jogging and beach volleyball she had enjoyed with her husband and friends. "I felt old and used up at 25," she sighed. "No wonder I was depressed."

Depression is a common side effect of osteoarthritis. It's natural to be upset as pain forces you to give up your favorite activities, makes routine chores difficult, and reminds you of its presence even when you're sitting down. The risk of depression rises as the pain becomes more severe and the disability increases, with unpredictable pain flare-ups making one feel like a hostage to the disease. Indeed, some researchers believe that loss of function or disability is even more likely to induce depression than is pain.[1] About 20 percent of osteoarthritis sufferers are depressed at any given time, a percentage consistent with the level of depression found among other groups of people with chronic diseases.[2]

What Is—and Is Not—Depression?

We commonly use the word *depression* to describe a large group of emotional disorders, ranging from mild to severe, that occur on a chronic, recurrent, or one-time-only basis.

Chronic depressive disorders may last for years or even decades, often with the symptoms striking most severely in the first two years. Recurrent depressive disorders will appear and disappear periodically, leaving one feeling healthy between episodes. And one-time-only bouts of depression may last for a few days or weeks, then vanish forever. If your doctor says that your depression is "clinical," it means that your symptoms are serious enough and/or frequent enough to warrant medical attention. There is also "subclinical" depression, a less severe version of the problem in which some symptoms are present, but they are not serious enough to lead to diagnosis or treatment. If the number of subclinical symptoms increases or if they become more severe, treatment may be warranted.[3]

Then there's the blues, otherwise known as "the blahs" or "feeling down in the dumps." This is *not* true depression. Instead, it's usually a reaction to an unpleasant event such as losing a job or failing a test. We feel bad for a while, then bounce back to our normal emotional states. Reacting to negative or stressful situations with the blues is perfectly normal. It only becomes a serious problem if it lasts for a significant period of time, if it is out of proportion to the unhappy situation, or if you feel you cannot shake the feeling on your own.

The Signs of Depression

It is perfectly normal to have *symptoms* of depression—we get them often. But if they don't seem to go away, if they get worse, or if more symptoms appear, you truly have the condition depression. Here's a list of problems to watch out for. If one or more of these lingers for weeks on end or longer, you may want to discuss the situation with your doctor:[4]

- loss of interest in the things you normally enjoy
- lack of interest in sex
- irritability or blue moods
- restlessness or a slowed-down feeling
- feelings of worthlessness or guilt
- appetite changes leading to weight gain or loss
- suicidal thoughts or thoughts of dying
- problems with concentration, thinking, or memory
- difficulty making decisions
- lack of sleep, or sleeping too much
- constant lack of energy
- headaches not caused by any other disease or condition
- other aches and pains not caused by any other disease or condition
- digestive problems unrelated to any other disease or condition
- feelings of hopelessness
- anxiety

- low self-esteem
- nightmares, especially with themes of loss, pain, or death
- preoccupation or obsession with failure, illness, or other unpleasant themes
- fear of being alone

An ongoing loss of interest in sex is an easy-to-spot symptom of depression among those who had previously enjoyed healthy sex lives. Pain, depression, fatigue, and stress can wreak havoc on your sex life, increasing your depression and feelings of hopelessness.

These are not the only symptoms of depression, and having one or more of these does not necessarily mean that you are clinically depressed. But they can point to problem areas. Your emotional health is as important as your physical health, so contact your doctor when you need help. (Don't use these guidelines for the purpose of self-diagnosis—only licensed and trained medical professionals are qualified to render a diagnosis.)

Who Is Most Likely to Become Depressed?

Doctors and psychologists have identified specific risk factors that increase the odds of depression. These apply to the general population, not just osteoarthritis sufferers. Your risk is increased if:[5]

————————◇————————

"KEEPING UP" AND "COVERING UP"

People with osteoarthritis have developed a variety of techniques to help them maintain their daily activities despite chronic pain. "Keeping up" occurs when you continue at your previous level of activity, despite increased pain or injury. You "keep up" because you want to prove that everything is okay. You may continue playing basketball on the weekends, or refuse work modifications that might make your job more manageable. It's possible for many people to "keep up" during the day, although they often suffer from excruciating pain and fatigue all evening and at night.

"Covering up" is an attempt to hide the osteoarthritis. You'll claim that you feel fine when people ask, even when you hurt. You'll refuse to use a cane, walker, or other device to assist you, because to do so would require you to acknowledge the pain. Instead of letting others see that you hurt, you may withdraw.

When "keeping up" or "covering up," you unwittingly cut off helpful support from your friends and loved ones, just when you need it most.[6]

————————◇————————

- You are a woman.
- You have already experienced a depressive event.
- Your first depressive event happened before age 40.
- You have a chronic medical condition or disease (including debilitating osteoarthritis).
- You have just had a baby.
- You have little or no emotional support (such as family and friends).
- You have just experienced a positive or negative stressful life event.
- You abuse drugs or alcohol.
- Your family has a history of depressive disorders.
- Earlier depressive events have only been partially relieved.
- You have attempted suicide.

You are not doomed to depression if you have one or more of these risk factors, and you are not guaranteed a depression-free life if you don't. However, this list of risk factors helps identify those who may be more susceptible to depression so they, their families, and physicians can watch for early signs of possible trouble.

If you have any sense that you may be depressed, get professional help *immediately*. Ask your doctor for a referral to a therapist. (If that doesn't work, ask a trusted friend or other health professional, such as a nurse.) Before your medical doctor refers you to a therapist, she or he should rule out the possibility of the depression being caused by a hormonal imbalance, Parkinson's disease, Huntington's disease, chronic fatigue syndrome, or other ailments. And since certain drugs can cause depression, your doctor should also ask you what medications you are currently or have recently been taking.

If you can't afford to pay for therapy, call your local mental health department to ask if they offer reduced-rate programs. You can also check with professional mental health organizations, osteoarthritis self-help groups, or your local chapter of the Arthritis Foundation.

If Your Osteoarthritis Has Left You Depressed . . .

Keep reminding yourself that your symptoms of depression will most likely vanish once the Arthritis Cure eliminates your pain and allows you to return to a normal life, but in the meantime . . .

Psychotherapy (the "talking cure") and drug therapy are the two major approaches to treating depression. Mild episodes of depression are usually treated with psychotherapy. In severe cases, drug therapy is often initiated immediately. The combined approach—psychotherapy and drug therapy—is becoming a popular treatment for most episodes of depression, even mild ones. The combined approach is being used more because:

• *It reestablishes normal body patterns more quickly.* Antidepressants can be used to normalize many of the problem areas affected by depression: sleep, appetite, sexual desire, and energy level. The sooner these areas return to normal states, the quicker the individual is on the road to full recovery.

• *It helps to ensure compliance in taking medications.* Doctors know that patients receiving help from psychotherapy are much more likely to take their medicines than those who do not have the additional support.

• *It recognizes the dual influence of biology and environment.* When researchers used PET (positron emission tomography) scans to create images of the brains of mentally ill patients, they observed that the use of medication and psychotherapy created identical changes in brain activity. In other words, psychotherapy and drug therapy influence the brain in similar ways. Using the two together is believed to be stronger than either one alone.

Be sure to check with your doctor before taking any medications to make sure you're not swallowing something that can aggravate your depression. Prednisone, indomethacin, and other painkillers used for osteoarthritis may cause depression. So can certain tranquilizers, including "downers" such as Valium and Librium. Codeine and other painkillers may cause or add to an existing depressive state. Sleeping pills may contribute to depression by altering your sleep patterns. That's why it's important to talk with your doctor *before* taking any medications.

Medicines Commonly Prescribed

Depression is a complex, mysterious syndrome, which is why developing medications to relieve its symptoms has been a complicated procedure. Today's antidepressant medications include several classes of drugs that can change the chemical activity of the brain. But they have differing effects on brain chemistry, which present a challenge to doctors prescribing them. Perhaps the biggest problem with antidepressants is their side effects, which can include dry mouth, nausea, diarrhea, headache, insomnia, jitteriness, dizziness, constipation, increased perspiration, appetite stimulation, anorexia, confusion, impotence, and, in men over 50, difficulty urinating. More severe complications include elevated blood pressure, irregular heartbeat, tremors, nausea, stroke, and anxiety. An overdose can lead to toxicity and possibly death.

Antidepressants also take a long time to work. Two, four, or up to eight weeks may pass before any positive changes are seen. And the initial improvements may be very subtle—a slightly more erect posture, smiling a little bit more, taking a little extra care about one's appearance. The patient's family often notices the changes before the patient does.[7]

Although medicines certainly have their place in treating depression, sometimes they just mask the symptoms, ignoring the underlying causes. And their side effects can be more dangerous than the original problem. Glucosamine and chondroitin, on the other hand, can be powerful "antidepressants," not because they work directly on one's mood, but because they help eliminate the underlying problem. But there is no such thing as an overnight miracle; it takes time for these two healing substances to work. That's why it's important to use a variety of depression-busting techniques. Some are stronger, some work faster, others last longer. Together, they can help to ensure recovery. And remember: If you are depressed because of osteoarthritis, your depression will likely clear up once the Arthritis Cure has gone to work.

Coping with Depression

If you become depressed because of restrictions osteoarthritis has placed on your life, learn how to cope. Mental health experts agree that those who cope best with disease are least likely to develop depression.[8] In other words, if you deal with your osteoarthritis, it's less likely to leave you depressed. Some of the best coping techniques are problem solving and flexibility. People who tackle their problems head on, coming up with creative solutions, do better. So do those who bend with the changes in their lives, adopting new activities, approaches, and ideas as they are forced to lay aside the old. For example, a creative, flexible person with osteoarthritis of the knee who can no longer jog for exercise may switch to swimming.

Joining a support group where you can find sympathetic ears and get some advice on coping is also a good idea. Each support group has a different tone, depending on the leader and the participants. Stay away from groups that spend too much time moaning and complaining. Instead, find one that emphasizes overcoming problems and getting on with your life. (You can find self-help groups by contacting the Arthritis Foundation.)

Beating Stress Helps Beat Depression

If osteoarthritis has made you depressed, take care to avoid as much stress as possible until you're feeling better, physically and emotionally. Stress is the response of the body, mind, and emotions to the everyday and extraordinary pressures of life. Stress is not the actual thing or event—it's our reaction. For example, being laid off from work may devastate one person, while another may find it an opportunity to find a better job or retire early. The situation is the same; it's the reaction that differs.

The fact that stress is the reaction, not the event itself, helps explain why some people are more stressed by their osteoarthritis than others. Some don't let their pain and disability bother them as much as others do. But even among those who take it relatively well, osteoarthritis can be a stressful event. Stress hits us in different ways, with symptoms that include:

- fatigue
- muscle tension
- anxiety
- irritability and anger
- upset stomach
- nervousness, trembling
- cold, sweaty hands
- loss or increase in appetite
- overall malaise (weakness, dizziness, headache, back pain, and other problems)

Stress may not *cause* depression, but it can certainly make it worse. It also signals certain glands to release high-voltage chemicals that can "shock" the body and weaken the immune system, making your osteoarthritis symptoms seem worse while increasing your risk of getting another disease.

The best defense against stress is a positive attitude. Remember, stress is not the event or thing—that's just the stressor. *How you respond to the stressor determines whether or not you're stressed.* This means that you can literally "think" stress away. Please understand: You are not responsible for being stressed; it's not your fault. However, by focusing on the problem you can increase your stress. The good news is that by focusing on all that is pleasant, optimistic, loving, helpful, and joyful, you can take a big bite out of stress. The unhappy event (your osteoarthritis) will still be there, but your re-

action to it will be different. Sure, arthritis is a pain.
But is it worth getting unduly upset about, if doing
so makes it worse? And yes, it's hard to smile in
the face of adversity. But if smiling makes it better,
then isn't smiling a medicine? That's why your prescription is to keep smiling, to fill your mind with
thoughts of love, joy, and optimism.

And while you're beating stress with a smile, you
can also build yourself up physically:

- Exercise regularly. Almost everyone can do some
  exercise, even those with severe osteoarthritis. If
  you can't jog anymore, try swimming. If aerobics
  class is too tough on your lower-body joints, try
  water aerobics or riding a stationary bike. Even if
  you're confined to bed, you can do strengthening
  exercises like leg lifts and upper-body work.
- Talk to your doctor about special exercises and
  activities that will help you maintain good posture and reduce stress on your joints.
- Give your body all the nutrients it needs by eating a healthful diet. Avoid sugar and caffeine,
  and stay away from fat and sugar-laden fast
  foods and desserts. Eat plenty of nutrient-rich
  fresh vegetables and fruits, plus whole grains.
- If you drink alcoholic beverages, do so in moderation. Stay away from drugs, unless they have
  been prescribed by your physician.
- Get plenty of sleep.
- Find a relaxation technique that works for you
  and practice it *daily*.

- Think of a way you can change your life for the better, then make that change.
- Learn to balance rest and activity—in other words, pace yourself.
- When you have a flare-up, modify your activities and take more time to rest.
- Don't overextend yourself, and plan ahead for a difficult task.
- Ask for help when you need it.
- Limit your activities and responsibilities to manageable levels.

Getting a Good Night's Sleep

Getting a good night's sleep is an excellent defense against stress, fatigue, and depression (unless your depression has prompted you to sleep too much). Here are some tips for better sleeping:

- Stick to a regular schedule of daily activity. Get up and go to bed at the same time each day.
- Exercise regularly, but not late at night.
- Create a quiet and comfortable environment in which to sleep. Get heavy curtains to block out light if it bothers you. If you're sensitive to noise, try a "white noise" machine that covers outside noises with the soothing sounds of a waterfall or waves on the beach.
- Spend an hour winding down before going to bed.

———————◇———————

GET TOUCHED

Touch is a powerful healing tool—its health-giving properties have been demonstrated over and over. Take newborn babies, for example. Studies comparing premature babies who are not touched with those who are gently touched have found that the "touched" babies gained 45 to 50 percent more weight before going home. The "touched" babies were more alert, active, and involved in their surroundings, and they went home earlier. The effects were lasting, for the "touched" babies tended to have fewer medical problems later in their young lives.[9]

Adults also benefit from being touched. Many medical scientists believe that touch can reduce psychological stress. And only a very soft touch is required—bear hugs are not a necessity. In fact, a bear hug may be too much for many osteoarthritis sufferers. A gentle, loving touch is a powerful medicine for everyone, one that can be very beneficial in fighting arthritis.

———————◇———————

- Take a relaxing bath before going to bed.
- Practice relaxation techniques.
- Listen to soothing music.
- Avoid caffeine in the evening.
- Beware of alcohol. A nightcap before bed can actually leave you feeling tired and unrested in the morning.

You **Can** *Overcome Depression*

Osteoarthritis can produce a host of psychological changes due to pain, frustration, depression, and stress. The Arthritis Cure tackles depression in two ways. First, glucosamine and chondroitin help by attacking the problem at the source—the osteoarthritis. Second, it gives you healthy mind and body techniques that are known to beat the blues. This two-pronged approach will help you overcome depression while regaining your emotional and physical health.

9

◊

You *Can* Prevent Osteoarthritis

This chapter will introduce you to the 7-step Osteoarthritis Prevention Program:

Eat a healthful, joint-preserving diet.

Maintain your ideal weight.

Exercise regularly.

Prevent injuries.

Ensure proper recovery if you are injured.

Optimize your biomechanics to counteract stress to your joints.

Consider use of glucosamine and chondroitin sulfates prophylactically.

◊

It's nice to know that the Arthritis Cure, spearheaded by glucosamine and chondroitin sulfates, can cure osteoarthritis once it has struck. But wouldn't it be even better to prevent the painful problem from rearing its ugly head in the first place?

We can. The 7-step Osteoarthritis Prevention Program can dramatically lower the risk of healthy joints suffering from osteoarthritic degeneration. It's impossible to absolutely guarantee that you will never be stricken by osteoarthritis, but we do know that the preventive program can work wonders. If you're reading this book, you probably already have osteoarthritis in at least one joint. You certainly don't want the other joints to suffer, so follow the prevention program to keep your other joints healthy, mobile, and pain-free. Once again, consult with your doctor before beginning this program.

The Osteoarthritis Prevention Program

You don't need high-tech medical instruments, highly paid specialists, exotic tests, or any other special tools to put the Osteoarthritis Prevention Program into action. All you need is some knowledge, a bit of time and thought, and determination to keep your joints healthy and strong. The prevention program is simple:

1. Eat a healthful, joint-preserving diet.
2. Maintain your ideal weight.
3. Exercise regularly.
4. Prevent injuries.
5. Ensure proper recovery if you are injured.
6. Optimize your biomechanics to counteract stress to your joints.
7. Consider use of glucosamine and chondroitin sulfates prophylactically, especially after injury.

That's all there is to it. And there are some great "side effects" to this program, such as dramatically reduced risks of having a heart attack or stroke, or of developing cancer and many other debilitating and possibly deadly diseases. You'll be putting yourself on the road to lifelong *great* health as you work to keep your joints strong and prevent ailments associated with painful joints.

Let's take a look at each of the seven points.

STEP 1 *Eat a Healthful Diet*

We've already looked at the diet that gives the body the nutritional tools it needs to build and maintain healthy joints. This same healthful diet can be used to prevent joint problems from occurring in the first place. Reread Chapter 7, and remember to:

• Balance your diet by eating the indicated amount of portions from each area.

• Limit your intake of fat. Not only does fat add calories to your diet and pounds to your waistline, but some fatty acids actually aggravate swelling and inflammation.[1] If you're an active person who sometimes gets a sprain or a strain, be especially aware of foods that might worsen the inflammation and encourage free radicals to further damage your joints.

• Eat foods containing antioxidants. Antioxidants counteract free radicals, those highly unstable molecules that can cause major damage to body tissues if left unchecked.[2] The antioxidants can also help to minimize tissue damage if you suffer a sprain or strain. Vitamins A, C, and E, plus the mineral selenium, are some of the many antioxidants found in most vegetables and fruits. (Free radicals have also been linked to cancer, heart disease, aging, and degenerative joint disease, so including antioxidants in your diet is an excellent all-around preventive measure.)

• Eat foods high in bioflavonoids. Bioflavonoids help to keep the collagen (an important part of the cartilage matrix) strong and resistant to inflammation. They also prevent free radical damage and help to heal damaged tissue following injury. Fortunately, the bioflavonoids are ubiquitous, meaning they're found in virtually all plant foods, including fresh vegetables, green tea, berries, onions, citrus fruits, and fruits that contain a pit (such as cherries and plums).[3]

• Eat foods that counter the harmful effects of medications. Certain drugs can drain important nutrients from your body. Common medicinal culprits include aspirin and NSAIDs, such as ibuprofen (e.g., Advil) or indomethacin (e.g., Indocin). These oft-prescribed drugs can alter your levels of iron, vitamin C, folic acid, and phosphorus, and decrease your body's ability to absorb these nutrients.[4] That's why it is very important to keep your vitamin levels high if you are taking any medication for an extended period of time.

STEP 2   *Maintain Ideal Body Weight*

Researchers at the Boston University Arthritis Center who studied the weight/osteoarthritis connection have concluded that weight loss can help to prevent the disease. They found that women who lost an average of eleven pounds over the ten-year study period were only about *half* as likely to develop osteoarthritis as those who weighed the same as or more than they did at the beginning of the study.[5]

It's clear that staying slim is a vital step in holding osteoarthritis at bay. Women are particularly susceptible to developing osteoarthritis when they are obese. But the clear message for both women and men of all ages: If you are carrying around too many pounds, get rid of them and you'll decrease your risk of osteoarthritis significantly. If you're already slim, stay that way.

STEP 3 *Exercise Regularly*

Proper exercise does to osteoarthritis what a daily apple does to the doctor: it keeps it away. Your preventive exercise program should be built on exercises that allow your joints to move painlessly through their natural rotation. For example, walking, rowing, swimming, cross-country skiing, and cycling help the knee and hip joints by keeping the joints moving and stimulating cartilage nourishment. Before becoming a marathon runner, rower, or cyclist, however, get yourself in good shape by gradually increasing your activities. And if you are overweight, your best bet is to begin with lower impact activities such as biking or brisk walking until you get closer to your ideal weight.

Remember that stretching and muscle conditioning are as important as aerobic conditioning. Stretching improves body awareness and makes your movements more graceful as it reduces the odds of certain kinds of injuries. It's also an effective antiaging tool. (Yoga is an excellent stretching exercise.) Strong muscles also play an important role in preventing osteoarthritis by supporting the joint area and absorbing shock. The muscles transfer weight away from the joint, thereby reducing the stress on the cartilage that comes with impact.

When choosing a type of anti-osteoarthritis exercise, select something you enjoy. There's much more to exercise than panting and sweating—it can and should be fun!

STEP 4   *Prevent Injuries*

Injuries are a common cause of *secondary osteoarthritis*. So whether you're an occasional exerciser, a dedicated athlete, or anything in between, take special care of injuries to your joints—and elsewhere. Sports that require pivoting, twisting, turning, and torquing into unnatural positions (such as soccer, football, skiing, basketball, volleyball, and tennis) are especially hard on the joints.[6]

Fortunately, many sports-related joint problems can be avoided if you take simple precautions. Start by getting and staying in good condition. Train before you play. Before hitting the slopes or stepping out on the tennis court, for example, exercise to build muscle strength around your joints and make your ligaments and tendons more resilient. Lifting weights three times a week during the "preseason" and once or twice a week when you're most active will help you keep up your strength. Stretch often, but only after you've warmed up. And be sure to balance your exercise program. Don't focus on just one group of muscles to the exclusion of others, for that can cause more problems later on.

Be sure to use the proper shoes and other equipment (pads, eye protection, helmets, and so on). The proper shoes absorb shock, support your arches, and prevent you from sliding while you play (which can put extra stress on the joints). Your shoes should correspond to the playing surface, so wear running shoes while running, tennis shoes for tennis, and so forth. Replace your shoes often, since worn-out shoes don't give you enough support or shock resistance.

Don't jump right into a high-level exercise program. Attempting to exercise like an Olympic athlete right off the bat can lead to injuries and frustration. Begin slowly, gradually increasing the level of difficulty/proficiency and the amount of time you spend exercising. If you wish to run, for example, it might be wise to start with brisk walking, followed by jogging several weeks later and eventually running (when you're in better shape). Doing drills specific to your sport is a great way to prevent injury. This prepares the body for the unpredictability of movements needed in play.

Warm up before you get out and do *anything*. A short, brisk walk or jog, or perhaps some jumping jacks and push-ups, will help loosen your muscles and get the blood flowing.

Be sure to cool down and stretch after every exercise session. Your muscles should be amenable to stretching now that they've been "warmed up." This is really the best time to increase your flexibility. Work on stretching several parts of your body, not just the muscles you use for your sport or exercise. And remember: avoid stretching a "cold" muscle, for that invites injury and does not usually lead to flexibility improvements.

Finally, get some training before you begin your new exercise or activity regimen. Don't just slap on the pads and start throwing body blocks; don't slide head first into home plate; don't put on the gloves and step into the boxing ring until you've learned exactly how it should be done. Even seemingly gentle sports like swimming and bicycling should be done properly in order to avoid injury. Technique is critical.

STEP 5 *Ensure Proper Recovery If You Are Injured*

If you do suffer an injury while exercising or participating in sports, make sure that you are completely recovered and rehabilitated *before* resuming your activity. Many active exercisers and athletes are inclined to downplay even serious injuries. How many times have we seen injured basketball or football players playing on tightly bandaged legs? Or a gymnast hurling over the vaulting horse despite an ankle injury? Stressing an already-injured joint can lead to long-term damage that is difficult or impossible to repair. That might be excusable at the Olympics, but why should the rest of us risk greater damage?

If you're injured, see your doctor. Get specific instructions as to how to care for your injury, and how long you should rest before starting up again. Your doctor may recommend that you take up a different activity to prevent future, irreversible damage.

Meanwhile, there are some simple steps you can follow for sprains or strains that you can still walk on or move with. Try the "RICE" approach[7]:

R—Rest your injured body part. Allowing damaged tissues to heal is critical. If you don't, you increase the risk of causing further damage by reinjuring the tissue.

I—Ice the injured area as soon as you can. This helps to reduce inflammation and swelling, both of which can slow down the healing process. Put a sock or thin towel between your skin and the ice, applying the ice for 20 minutes three times a day for a few days.

C—Compress the injured area with an Ace bandage or other restrictive device to prevent swelling. If you use an Ace bandage, be careful not to wrap it so tightly that it restricts blood flow. (You should be able to easily slip a finger underneath the bandage.) If your skin starts to discolor, or if the area below the bandage starts to swell, the bandage is too tight.

E—Elevate the injured body part to help prevent swelling. This also forces you to rest the injured area. If you are lying down, elevate the injured area so that it is higher than your heart.

Once the pain and inflammation are under control, you can start working on rehabilitating the injured area, regaining flexibility and strength. Give your body enough time to rest and recover, to gain back strength and flexibility before pulling on your sweats and "getting out there" again. It's better to wait a little longer, rather than risk reinjury.

*   *   *

Beware: If you are experiencing severe or unusual pain, if you hear or feel something "pop," if you have a deformity, or if anything else seems amiss, see your doctor or go to an emergency room right away.

STEP 6   *Optimize Your Biomechanics to Counteract Stress to Your Joints*

The same biomechanical techniques that help treat osteoarthritis can be used to prevent the disease. Many people unknowingly walk, jump, swing a tennis racquet, or otherwise move in ways that place unnatural stress on their joints. A biomechanical evaluation can detect and set you on the road to correcting these movement "glitches" before they cause serious trouble.

STEP 7   *Consider Use of Glucosamine and Chondroitin Sulfates Prophylactically*

If you have a higher-than-average risk of developing osteoarthritis, but are not yet suffering symptoms, you may help head off trouble by using glucosamine and chondroitin sulfates on a preventive basis. (Studies are currently under way to determine who would best benefit from prophylactic use of glucosamine and chondroitin sulfates for arthritis prevention.) Since there are no known significant side effects, even over the long term, the potential risks from taking these two supplements is lower than the risks of swallowing a daily aspirin. And to our knowledge, clinical studies have found no significant long-term side effects.

How do you know if your risk is higher than average? Do you fit into any of the following categories?

• *You have a genetic predisposition.* Certain forms of osteoarthritis appear to be inherited. The most common type is *primary generalized osteoarthritis*, in which three or more joints are affected for no known reason. Heberden's nodes and Bouchard's nodes are common in those with a genetic predisposition. A second type of inherited osteoarthritis is associated with *familial chondrocalcinosis*, a disease in which calcium crystals are deposited in cartilage. Then there's *Stickler Syndrome*, also known as hereditary arthro-ophthalmopathy, which occurs in about 1 out of every 10,000 people and is characterized by vision problems (usually shortsightedness) and premature degenerative joint disease.

• *You're obese.* In women especially, being obese is a risk for getting osteoarthritis, and losing weight can dramatically reduce the risk. Obesity in this context is defined using body mass index (BMI). The BMI is the weight (in kilograms) divided by the square of height (in meters). Values above 25 characterize obesity. So, if you are five feet tall and weight over 128 pounds, your BMI is over 25. The same holds true for those five feet six and over 155 pounds, or if you're six feet tall and above 184 pounds. Dropping two BMI units decreases knee osteoarthritis risk by over 50 percent in women.[8,9] The link between obesity and knee osteoarthritis has been well established. Obese women are prime candidates for this arthritis.

• *You have suffered a major trauma or sports injury to a joint.*

• *You engage in repetitive impact loading activities.* Ballet dancers, pneumatic drill operators, baseball pitchers, and others who engage in certain repetitive motions are at high risk, especially if they use their joints in unintended ways.

• *You have misaligned bones.* Bone misalignment can lead to unusual stress on the joint and osteoarthritis. This is actually very common in the hips and can lead to early arthritis with no other apparent cause.

If you belong to any of the risk groups, you may want to consider preventive glucosamine and chondroitin therapy.

Summing Up

Here's the Osteoarthritis Prevention Program:

1. Eat a healthful, joint-building diet.
2. Maintain your ideal weight.
3. Exercise regularly.
4. Prevent injuries.
5. Ensure proper recovery if you are injured.

6. Optimize your biomechanics to counteract stress to your joints.
7. Consider use of glucosamine and chondroitin sulfates prophylactically.

It's simple, inexpensive and easy to follow. All you have to do is decide to do it, and you're already on your way to reducing your risk of osteoarthritis while improving your overall health. And be sure to discuss this program with your doctor before starting.

10

Rheumatic Disease Review

The most common forms of arthritis.

Other diseases that affect the joints.

◇

Some people mix up osteoarthritis and rheumatoid arthritis, two very different rheumatologic diseases with similar names. And it gets even more confusing when you learn that there are more than *100 different types* of rheumatic diseases, many causing different forms of arthritis. Depending upon the type of arthritis, the associated inflammation may flare up in one joint or many, may limit itself to the joint only, or might spread to the muscles, tendons, ligaments, internal organs, and even the skin. Different types of arthritis have different causes, courses, and cures.

Naturally, your arthritis cannot be effectively treated until the type has been diagnosed. Your doctor will make the diagnosis, which may very well be one of these common forms:

ANKYLOSING SPONDYLITIS

If you wake up in the morning with lower back pain and stiffness, if sitting or lying down for more than a couple of hours makes your back feel worse, if your chest hurts when you inhale, and if you're tired and losing weight, you may be suffering from ankylosing spondylitis (AS).

Causing bent or fused spinal vertebrae, AS is most commonly seen in young men. It sometimes goes untreated in earlier stages because it can easily be confused with mechanical back pain, the kind you get from lifting a heavy object. With AS, the tendons and ligaments that make it possible to move the back become inflamed. The vertebrae respond to the problem by producing more bone. The body's response is well intentioned, but making extra bone can cause the vertebrae to grow into each other and fuse together. Eventually, the spine can wind up looking like a bamboo pole, and it bends forward under the weight of the head. If you have ever seen an elderly person walking bent over as though he were looking at his shoes, you have probably witnessed the late stages of AS.

AS inflammation usually begins in the lower back, and almost always involves the sacroiliac joints (the joints where the lower spine meets the pelvis). In later stages the middle and upper back are afflicted. The disease can spread down into the buttocks and thighs, or up into the chest, where it can make deep breathing painful. The inflammation may also strike the joints of the shoulders, knees, or ankles. In fact, in some 20 percent of AS cases the first signs of arthritis appear in the shoulder, hips, or other joints. But most of the time the disease is confined to the lower back and is relatively mild. People with AS are not usually disabled and don't have shortened careers or life spans.

Young men between 16 and 35 years of age are the favorite targets of AS, which afflicts approximately 1 in 1,000 people under the age of 40. Three times as many males as females are diagnosed with the disease, but this may be because females tend to have much milder symptoms and may never be diagnosed. It also appears in children (mostly boys), who account for roughly 5 percent of the cases. It is rarely seen in African-Americans.

Scientists have found what may prove to be a genetic basis for AS. The disease is found almost exclusively in those who have the HLA-B27 gene, a gene involved in fighting infection. But don't worry if you have HLA-B27, for only 20 percent of those with the gene eventually develop the disease. It's not enough to have the genetic tendency; the gene has to be "switched on" somehow. (If one identical twin develops AS, it appears in the other twin only 60 percent of the time.) Studies currently under way are looking into the possibility that a certain type of infection triggers AS.

Early diagnosis and proper treatment of AS can reduce or prevent deformity. The treatment regimens are designed to reduce pain and prevent deformities while strengthening the back and neck. Nonsteroidal anti-inflammatory drugs (NSAIDs) are used to reduce pain and inflammation, although for some reason aspirin doesn't seem to provide much relief. Exercise and posture improvement help to increase strength and flexibility, while minimizing deformity. AS victims are often taught to sleep on their stomachs to help keep their backs from curving forward.[1, 2, 3]

BURSITIS AND TENDINITIS

Many an unhappy weekend athlete is familiar with bursitis and tendinitis, that pain and tenderness in the shoulders, elbows, knees, or pelvis that radiates into the nearby limbs, and is sometimes accompanied by fever. "B&T" are the most common forms of soft tissue rheumatic syndromes. They're usually caused by sudden overuse of a joint. It's the areas around the joints of the shoulders, elbows, wrists, fingers, hips, back, knees, ankles, and feet that often pay the price for the overenthusiastic use.

Bursa means *purse*, and the small fluid-filled sacs (bursae) that cushion various parts of the joints do look something like little purses. There are dozens of them in the body; each knee has eight or more. The bursae, which act as cushions (usually between soft tissue and a bony prominence), may become inflamed if a joint is subjected to abnormal pressure. This is most often the result of overuse or of a chronic condition or a trauma such as a fall on the knee or elbow. The bursae can fill with more fluid than usual, triggering pain. Common forms of bursitis are "housemaid's knee" and "student's elbow," which are both caused by leaning too long or too heavily on a joint.

Tendinitis is often grouped with bursitis, but is a very different problem. Tendinitis is characterized by the inflammation or irritation of a tendon, that tough, fibrous many-layered tissue that ties muscles to bones. We normally think that bones move only when muscles contract, but remember that the tendon is "between" the muscle and the bone, allowing the two to work together. Contracting a muscle to move a bone means that the tendons automatically "move" as well. Forcing swollen tendons to move, however, can be quite painful. Tendinitis is a risk factor for tendon rupture, especially when engaging in ballistic activities (fast takeoffs or jumping).

Tendinitis usually strikes suddenly. It's usually localized (restricted to one area), and can linger for days or weeks before disappearing. Many of us will have tendinitis at one time or another in our lives, but fortunately, permanent damage or disability from this condition is rare. It may strike the outside of the elbow as "tennis elbow," the inside of the elbow as "golfer's elbow," the tendons that move the fingers as "trigger finger," the bottom of the pelvis as "weaver's bottom," the finger joints as "video game finger," or the wrist and base of the thumb as deQuervain's tendinitis.

Bursitis and tendinitis usually occur after age 30, the result of wear and tear on the bursae and/or tendons, abnormal stress on joints or tendons, overly ambitious workouts by "weekend warriors," or a sudden strain, such as lifting a heavy package. "B&T" are usually not chronic conditions, and permanent damage is rare. (Recurring tendinitis can be a sign of ankylosing spondylitis, however, so see your doctor.)

Treatment of bursitis and tendinitis occurs in phases. Phase I is to remove the aggravating factor(s), use ice, massage, take NSAIDs as appropriate, and do some gentle stretching and range-of-motion exercises. Phase II adds physical therapy such as ultrasound or electric stimulation, plus supervised strengthening exercises and moving of the surrounding structures. Phase III brings into play injections of NSAIDs or a cortisonelike drug. Phase IV is surgery, which is rarely needed and only used if the first three phases do not help after several months.[4, 5, 6]

GOUT

When someone mentions gout, we usually think of the huge-bellied, gluttonous King Henry VIII swilling port wine and chewing on a leg of mutton, his bandaged foot resting on a stool. Gout was once called the "rich man's disease" because it was associated with being overweight, overeating (especially of meats), and overindulging in drink. Today we know that gout is a metabolic disorder, but a poor diet can make the condition worse.

In gout, uric acid, a waste product in the urea (urine) cycle, is either overproduced, underexcreted, or both. When a person has too much uric acid in his or her system, some of it forms uric acid crystals. These crystals (think of them as sharp pieces of glass inside your body) can be deposited into the joint space, rather than being cleared by the kidneys. These "glass shards" often find their way to the "bunion joint" of the big toe, although gout is also found in the other joints of the feet, as well as those of the fingers, wrists, elbows, knees, and ankles. The afflicted joint suddenly becomes hot, painfully swollen, and stiff; fever and chills sometimes follow. The skin of the affected area can appear shiny red or purple, and pain from an acute attack of gout can be excruciating. In some cases, the joint is so tender that the light brush of a bed sheet can cause howls of pain.

Gout affects about two million Americans, most of them male (80 percent). Risk factors for getting the disease include a family history of gout, drinking alcohol, high blood pressure, taking certain medications, being overweight, or gaining weight. Unchecked, gout can be hazardous to your health, for the uric acid crystals may eventually be deposited in the soft tissue, cartilage, joints, tendons, or elsewhere, forming lumps. The crystals can also damage the kidneys. The good news is that gout can often be completely controlled with proper treatment, which usually includes the use of non-steroidal anti-inflammatory drugs (NSAIDs) for pain and inflammation, abstinence from alcohol, dietary restrictions, and possibly medications to reduce the amount of uric acid production or increase its excretion.[7, 8, 9]

INFECTIOUS ARTHRITIS

Can arthritis be brought about by "germs"? Absolutely. Many forms of bacteria, viruses, and fungi can cause infectious arthritis, which is frequently characterized by loss of joint function, fever, and inflammation of one or more joints and (occasionally) chills. The knee is most commonly involved (50 percent of the cases), followed by the hip, shoulder, wrist, and ankle. Infectious arthritis can generally be cured if caught early enough.

Practically any bacterium, virus, or fungus that produces disease can prompt this infectious form of arthritis, and there are many ways that the infecting agent can enter the body: trauma, surgery, inserting a needle into a joint, abscess or bone infection near the joint, animal bites, insect bites (Lyme disease), and even thorns. A less obvious but common source of joint infection is bacteria from a distant site in the body that travels through the bloodstream before settling in a joint. Infections almost anywhere in the body can move to the joints, including infections that begin in the lungs, urinary tract, and skin. Remember that any invasive procedure involving a joint (surgery, injection into the joint space) can lead to infection and infectious arthritis. This is an important consideration when opting for certain arthritis treatments that involve injecting medicine directly into the joint.

The body responds to the infection by mobilizing the immune system and engaging in a fierce battle with the infectious agent. The joint becomes the battleground. Like all battlegrounds, the joint suffers, becoming inflamed and painful as the body releases enzymes that inadvertently degrade the cartilage as they seek to destroy the invaders. Chronic alcoholics and drug abusers are at high risk for infectious arthritis, as are those suffering from diabetes, sickle cell anemia, kidney disease, and certain forms of cancer.

The goal in treating infectious arthritis is first to eliminate the infection, then handle the arthritis itself. Treatment depends upon what caused it in the first place: antibiotics are prescribed for bacterial causes, while NSAIDs are the medicine of choice for viral causes. Infected joints may be drained in order to allow the medication to act more effectively. In the early stages of treatment, resting splints are often used to limit the movement of joint tissue. Physical therapy may then be used to build up muscle strength and relieve joint stiffness.[10, 11]

JUVENILE ARTHRITIS

A temperature that swings up and down on a daily basis, chills, possibly a body rash, plus pain or swelling in the toes, knees, ankles, elbows, or shoulders are the hallmarks of juvenile arthritis.

Juvenile arthritis is a general term for the various kinds of arthritis that can strike children under the age of 16. The most common form that children in the United States suffer from is juvenile rheumatoid arthritis (JRA). JRA appears in three distinct forms: *systemic*, *polyarticular*, and *pauciarticular*, with the common characteristics of joint inflammation (stiffness, swelling, pain, warmth, and redness).

In *systemic JRA* (also known as Still's disease), there is usually a fever of 103 or more, which disappears in a few hours, only to reappear the next day. This high temperature may be accompanied by shaking chills, swollen lymph nodes, and a rash with a peculiar salmon-pink color. These signs and symptoms may last for weeks or even months. Many joints can be affected, as well as the blood and the outer lining of the heart or lungs. There may be stomach pain, severe anemia, and a high white cell count. Systemic JRA should always be closely monitored by a physician.

Polyarticular JRA appears in several joints (five or more). Like rheumatoid arthritis, it often strikes symmetrically, affecting the same joint on both sides of the body (such as both knees). In some cases, the patient may also suffer a slight fever and eye inflammation. Girls are more likely to contract this long-term disease, which can extend into adulthood and is thought to be the same as adult rheumatoid arthritis. Another type of polyarticular JRA seems to strike mostly boys. This form is characterized by stiffness in the hips and lower back, with arthritis in the large joints, and often develops into ankylosing spondylitis as the child reaches adulthood.

Pauciarticular JRA affects only a few joints, most often the large ones such as the knee, ankle, or elbow. It is not usually symmetrical.

Because of the pain, children with arthritis tend to avoid moving their inflamed joints. As a result, the unused joints can become chronically stiff and the surrounding muscles weak. In rare instances, long-term inflammation can damage the joint surfaces, causing deformity.

We don't know what causes JRA. However, it is not contagious and rarely appears in more than one child in a family. The disease is usually treated with aspirin and other NSAIDs, and sometimes gold treatment injections. In severe cases, low doses of corticosteroids may be prescribed. Exercise helps to prevent stiffness and maintain muscle strength, and surgery may be necessary to correct severe joint damage.[12, 13]

PSEUDOGOUT

The name makes it sound as if it's a fake, but the pain and other symptoms of pseudogout are real. Often striking the knee joint, then the wrists and ankles, pseudogout attacks suddenly, causing pain and swelling in the joint and possibly destroying cartilage. An attack may go on for days or weeks, with the acute phase lasting 12 to 36 hours. Or the pain may flare up in several joints at a time, though it is usually less severe and more chronic. Sometimes the pain increases after activity; sometimes it doesn't. These symptoms often disappear without treatment.

Also known as calcium pyrophosphate dihydrate crystal deposition disease, pseudogout has only recently been recognized as a form of arthritis. As is the case with gout, the pain is caused by crystals deposited in the joint spaces, but in pseudogout the crystals are formed from calcium pyrophosphate rather than uric acid. These calcium crystals can also be deposited into the cartilage, causing a condition called chondro-calcinosis (Latin for "calcium in the cartilage").

Pseudogout usually doesn't appear before the age of 65 (rarely is it seen in anyone under 30), and it seems to affect men and women equally. The disease can be brought on by surgery, trauma, or stress, but not by diet. Even though the crystals contain calcium, drinking milk or eating high-calcium foods doesn't seem to make a difference.

Treatment includes joint aspiration to remove the fluid containing the crystals, NSAIDs to manage pain and inflammation, plus rest and/or splints during an acute attack to protect the joints. Exercise helps to build muscle strength and restore full motion of the joints after an acute attack. In rare instances, surgery may be used to replace a joint that has been badly damaged, is extremely painful, or is unstable.[14, 15]

PSORIATIC ARTHRITIS
An inherited disease, this form of arthritis sometimes occurs in people with the skin condition called psoriasis. Psoriasis causes red, scaly patches that often appear on the neck, knees, and elbows, and the nails may become pitted. Psoriatic arthritis can settle in the end joints of the fingers or toes, causing them to become so swollen that they're often referred to as "sausage digits."

The joints in the extremities are most often affected, and the diagnosis can't be made unless the patient has skin and nail involvement consistent with psoriasis. Although the disease is chronic, most people with psoriatic arthritis feel well, with the exception of their joint pain. They generally don't suffer from fatigue or bone weakening.

Psoriatic arthritis usually appears when its victims are between the ages of 20 and 30, although it may occur at any age. It affects men and women equally, and occurs in 5 to 8 percent of those who have psoriasis. Treatment regimens include NSAIDs to reduce the inflammation, exercises to improve joint mobility, and rest. In a small number of cases, methotrexate is prescribed. Gold injections have sometimes been effective.[16, 17, 18]

REITER'S SYNDROME

First described by Dr. Hans Reiter during World War I, Reiter's syndrome is a disease that affects the joints, eyes, skin, and urinary tract. Reiter's is an "itis" disease (*itis* means *inflammation*) characterized by arthritis and at least two of the following:

urethritis (inflammation of the urethra)
prostatitis (inflammation of the prostate gland)
stomatitis (painless mouth ulcers)
conjunctivitis ("pinkeye")
dermatitis (scaly skin rash, especially on the
   penis)

The many symptoms of Reiter's include inflammation of the urethra (the tube carrying urine out of the body), the urge to urinate frequently, a low fever, redness of the eyes, an unpleasant discharge within two weeks after sexual intercourse, plus skin lesions around the fingernails, toenails, and on the palms of the hands or soles of the feet. There may also be pain in the joints, especially in the back, hips, legs, and toes. Not all patients have all of these signs and symptoms.

The cause of Reiter's syndrome is unknown. There appears to be a genetic predisposition to the disease, but the "trigger" may be an infection transmitted sexually or through the gastrointestinal tract.

Men between the ages of 20 and 40 are the primary victims of Reiter's syndrome. Women also get the disease, but men are more likely to be diagnosed because their symptoms are more obvious. Treatment regimens consist of NSAIDs to reduce the pain and inflammation, and antibiotics if the triggering infection is known. Doctors also strongly recommend that men with Reiter's syndrome use condoms to avoid spreading the disease if the infection has not yet been treated.[19, 20, 21]

RHEUMATOID ARTHRITIS (RA)

RA is an autoimmune disease brought about when the body has "turned on itself," with the immune system attacking bodily tissues just as if they were foreign invaders. In its mildest form, rheumatoid arthritis is characterized by joint discomfort; in its most serious form it can cause painfully deformed joints and harm organ systems.

Some experts believe that RA is brought about by a bacterial infection in the joints. It might also be triggered by a virus settling in those who are genetically susceptible, causing the joint lining (especially the part that meets the cartilage) to become inflamed. Over time, chronic inflammation makes the joint lining thick and overgrown. This overgrown lining may then start to invade the cartilage, other joint-supporting tissues, and even the bone, weakening the entire joint structure. Eventually, the weakened joint becomes more painful and less able to perform. Under pressure, it may even become dislocated and deformed.

Usually appearing in the same joint on both sides of the body (both hands, for example), RA hits suddenly. The joints become swollen, tender, and inflamed. There may also be fever, weight loss, and a general feeling of sickness, soreness, stiffness, and aching. The eyes and mouth may dry out if the tear and salivary glands become involved.

RA affects more than two million people in the United States, striking women three times as often as men. Onset is typically between the ages of 20 and 40, although older persons and children are also victims. About 10 percent of those affected with the disease have a single episode followed by a spontaneous long-term remission. For the other 90 percent, joint inflammation is chronic, although mild, with occasional attacks or "flares." The disease may get progressively worse over time.

The treatment for RA is designed to alleviate pain, reduce inflammation, stop or slow joint damage, and improve overall body functioning. Aspirin and NSAIDs are employed as a first line of defense, with limited doses of corticosteroids sometimes used. Other treatments include injectable gold salts and methotrexate. Exercise and therapy can help reduce joint stiffness and swelling, alleviate pain, and increase joint mobility. Surgery is an option in the case of severe damage to the hips or knees and sometimes the shoulder when it can make the difference between dependence and independence.[22, 23, 24, 25]

Other Diseases That Affect the Joints

Arthritis is not the only disease that attacks the joints. Other diseases, arising in various parts of the body, may damage the joints as a side effect. The following diseases are not truly forms of arthritis, but they can cause arthritis-like symptoms.

FIBROMYALGIA

Characterized by widespread, possibly incapacitating pain, fibromyalgia produces stiffness and weakness of the muscular areas of the lower back, hips, thighs, neck, shoulder, chest, or arms, accompanied by muscle spasms ("Charley horses") in any of those areas. Patients often tell their doctors: "I hurt all over." The symptoms of fibromyalgia are quite similar to those of chronic fatigue syndrome, which explains why doctors have had a hard time distinguishing between the two. But in recent years, researchers have discovered that the diagnosis of fibromyalgia is based on pain or tenderness in at least 11 of 18 specific points of the body.

Formerly referred to as fibrositis, fibromyalgia literally means "muscle pain." When the disease strikes, the connective tissue layers of the muscles, tendons, and bones become inflamed. Chronic pain (described as burning, radiating, gnawing, or aching) may begin in one area of the body, such as the neck, then spread to other areas. But the stiffness and tenderness centers in the ligaments, tendons, and muscles rather than in the joints (as it would with arthritis). That's why fibromyalgia is considered a "soft tissue syndrome" rather than a true arthritis.

Women between the ages of 35 and 60 are the most likely victims of fibromyalgia, with the highest incidence occurring just before menopause. No specific cause has been pinpointed, and it is often misdiagnosed because most of its symptoms are similar to those found in other conditions.

Treatment of fibromyalgia includes alleviating chronic pain and sleep disturbances, as well as dealing with the depression that often accompanies a chronic disease. Water exercises, biofeedback, and relaxation techniques are all helpful. Although aspirin and NSAIDs are usually prescribed to relieve the pain, they don't always do the job. That's why muscle relaxants or local anesthetics are sometimes injected into the painful areas to quickly relax the muscle and alleviate pain.[26, 27, 28]

PAGET'S DISEASE

Also known as osteitis deformans, Paget's disease is a bone disorder characterized by bone pain and deformity. With the disease, the normal process of bone remodeling (breakdown and build-up) speeds up markedly. New, bulkier, and softer bone is produced, but it's weaker and has a greater tendency to fracture than normal bone. Paget's disease most often strikes the bones of the pelvis, skull, spine, and the long bones of the leg. The weakened bone structure characteristic of the disease leads to arthritis in the nearby joints. Ringing in the ears and hearing loss may occur if the small bones of the ear have been targeted by the disease. The rapid bone formation gradually stops. The symptoms may appear and disappear, but any bone alteration or damage that has already occurred is permanent.

There are usually no symptoms at onset, so the early presence of the disease can only be detected by routine blood tests. When symptoms do arise, they can best be described as "deep bone pain," a feeling of warmth all over, or headaches if the skull bones are affected. Bones are chronically painful (especially at night); they seem to be getting larger and the skin that covers them feels unusually warm. Bone formation is altered as the disease progresses, causing a weakening, thickening, and deformity of the bones. Movement may be impaired, and the bones may fracture easily.

Paget's disease is more common in men than women, and often surfaces between the ages of 50 and 70. It may run in families, and most of those affected are Caucasians of northwestern European ancestry (although the disease is occasionally seen in African-Americans). The cause of Paget's is unknown. Treatment centers on relieving pain, preventing bone deformity or fracture, and protecting hearing. A medication used for osteoporosis, Fosamax (alendronate) is also given to patients with Paget's disease. Surgery may be used to correct both hearing loss and bowed bones.[29, 30]

POLYMYALGIA RHEUMATICA (PMR)

PMR is a condition characterized by stiffness and aching originating in the muscles of the neck, shoulder, and hips, especially in the morning. Patients often complain that they just can't get out of bed in the morning due to their stiffness. The disease hits rapidly: a full set of symptoms can appear in one day, including pain in the jaw muscles when eating or talking, severe headaches, tenderness of the scalp or temples, hearing difficulties, a persistent sore throat, swallowing difficulties, and cough. In rare instances the blood supply to an eye may be affected, leading to blindness in that eye. It is uncertain as to whether or not PMR involves the joints, muscles, or arteries, and its cause is unknown. Corticosteroids, the standard treatment for PMR, are usually effective, but they have their side effects.[31, 32, 33]

POLYMYOSITIS AND DERMATOMYOSITIS

Commonly referred to as *myositis*, these two diseases are characterized by inflammation of the connective tissues, with weakening and subsequent breakdown of the muscles (polymyositis) and skin (dermatomyositis).

Polymyositis produces an inflammation of the muscle (especially in the arms and legs) that leads to the destruction of muscle fiber and wasting-away of the muscle. If the shoulder is involved, the victim will have difficulty reaching up to comb his or her hair or to take a dish out of the cupboard. If muscles in the hip area are attacked, it may become difficult for a person to get out of a chair or climb stairs. In its most severe form, polymyositis can weaken muscles in the neck and throat, changing the voice and making it difficult to swallow. If chest muscles are affected, it may become hard to breathe.

With dermatomyositis, a reddish patchy rash can appear on the face, knuckles, elbows, knees, ankles, or around the eyes. Sometimes the eyelids will become puffy and have a purplish color. In the more advanced cases, rubbing a finger across the affected area can take off several layers of skin.

Other symptoms of polymyositis and dermato-myositis include fever, weight loss, and joint pain. No one knows exactly what causes myositis, although it has many similarities to lupus and rheumatoid arthritis and is probably the result of hypersensitivity or autoimmune problems. Myositis appears gradually over a period of months. It usually strikes when one is between the ages of 30 and 60, and affects twice as many women as men. Most patients respond well to treatment, although

can be fatal in some, including older people who
lso have cancer.[34, 35, 36]

Myositis is treated with corticosteroids for the
uscle weakness, plus physical therapy. Rest is
lso important, especially during the acute stage.

CLERODERMA

cleroderma means "thick skin," so it's no wonder
hat the disease is characterized by a hardening and
ickening of the skin on the hands, arms, and face,
s well as ulcers on the fingers, hair loss, and skin
iscoloration. It also affects the joints, blood ves-
els, and internal organs.

The body's tiny blood vessels and capillaries be-
ome inflamed when scleroderma strikes, prompt-
ig the body to overproduce collagen. The excess
ollagen is deposited in the skin and body organs
here it hardens, causing the skin to thicken and
e internal organs to malfunction. Although the
ints themselves aren't damaged by scleroderma,
ey may feel stiff because the skin has become
ard. Indeed, the fingers may become stiff and
awlike as excess cartilage is deposited, even
ough the joints themselves are still healthy. The
ost severe complications of the disease are related
the deposition of collagen and consequent scar-
ng of the internal organs. Scleroderma induced
amage to the esophagus, heart, lungs, kidneys, or
testinal tract can be fatal.

Women are affected by scleroderma five times
ore often than men. The disease's favorite targets
e women between the ages of 30 and 60, although

it can strike either sex at any age. Like rheumatoid arthritis, scleroderma is believed to be an autoimmune disease triggered by an unknown factor. The trigger may be environmental or chemical (sclerodermalike diseases have been seen in workers who are exposed to silica dust or vinyl chloride, as well as in people taking the cancer drug bleomycin or the amino acid supplement L-tryptophan.) Patients receiving bone marrow transplants sometimes develop a condition that closely resembles scleroderma.

There is no cure for scleroderma, but several medications are used to control the symptoms. These include aspirin and NSAIDs for pain and inflammation, corticosteroids for muscle problems, antacids for heartburn, and medications to control high blood pressure and stimulate circulation. Careful exercise helps to maintain overall fitness and to keep the skin and joints flexible. Protecting the skin from further damage is also an important part of the treatment of scleroderma.[37, 38, 39]

SJÖGREN'S SYNDROME

After rheumatoid arthritis, Sjögren's is the most common autoimmune rheumatic disease. It inflames the tear and saliva glands, causing dry eyes and mouth. Itchy, red, irritated eyes and cloudy vision are common symptoms, as well as cracks in the tongue or at the corners of the mouth, difficulty chewing and swallowing, and a decreased sense of taste. Other problems associated with Sjögren' syndrome include rampant dental caries, joint in flammation, inflammation of the lungs, kidneys, liver, nerves, thyroid glands, and brain, and fatigue. A mild form of arthritis usually accompanies the condition.

Sjögren's syndrome is an autoimmune disease often found in conjunction with lupus, rheumatoid arthritis, or scleroderma. Although no specific cause has been determined, it is believed that heredity, viral infections, and hormones may be important factors in the disease. Sjögren's can strike anyone at any time, but 90 percent of those who get it are women, and it is rare among those under the age of 20.

Treatment is designed to relieve discomfort while controlling mouth and eye dryness. Lubricating eye drops, chewing gum, and room humidifiers may be helpful. Aspirin and NSAIDs are used to reduce joint pain, inflammation, and muscle aches. Exercise can help to keep joints and muscles flexible.[40, 41]

SYSTEMIC LUPUS ERYTHEMATOSUS

Also known as lupus or SLE, this autoimmune disease attacks and inflames connective tissues throughout the body. Its victims may have a red rash spread across the bridge of their noses and cheeks. The rash resembles markings on wolves, which explains the name of the disease (*lupus* is Latin for *wolf*).

Affecting nine times as many women as men, lupus usually strikes during the childbearing years (18 to 45) and is found in about 1 out of 2,000 people. The disease causes the production of abnormal antibodies called antinuclear antibodies (ANA) that damage bodily tissues. The skin, kidneys, nervous system, muscles, lungs, and heart can all be affected, as well as the joints (especially the fingers, wrists, and knees). Besides the red rash on the face, common symptoms include joint pain, stiffness, fever, muscle ache, weight loss, loss of hair, and exhaustion. There may also be a sensitivity to ultraviolet light, with exposure to the sun worsening the rash. As the disease progresses, inflammation of the linings of the heart, lungs, and kidneys can cause permanent damage.

As with scleroderma and rheumatoid arthritis, an unknown trigger may set lupus in motion, but only in those who are already genetically susceptible. It occurs more often in African-Americans than it does in Caucasians, and some data suggest that Asian and Hispanic populations also have a higher incidence than Caucasians. Some lupus patients have also been found to be lacking in a certain enzyme involved in healthy immune responses, and thus may be more likely to fall victim to the disease.

The degree of severity of the disease varies quite a bit from person to person. Some don't even know they have it and require no treatment at all, while for others it is a major illness. The majority of people, however, have moderate symptoms and function quite well.

The treatment of lupus includes aspirin and other NSAIDs for pain and inflammation, antimalarial drugs for active attacks or when an extensive rash is present, ointments or skin creams to treat the rashes, and corticosteroids in severe cases (especially if the kidneys are affected). Exercise, avoiding excessive sun exposure, and resting during the active stages of the disease are also important. And patients may need to avoid certain chemicals such as hair spray, paints, insecticides, and fertilizers that seem to trigger acute attacks.[42, 43, 44, 45]

TEMPORAL ARTERITIS (TA)

Temporal arteritis is an inflammatory disease of the large arteries in the head, neck, and elsewhere in the body. Its symptoms include pain, aching, and stiffness in the muscles of the upper arms, trunk, and legs (particularly in the morning), a headache that usually pounds away in one temple, tenderness, swelling, and redness following the path of the temporal artery on one side of the head, mild fever, and loss of appetite. TA affects the arteries, preventing them from delivering an adequate blood supply to the connective tissues. The collagen is adversely affected, which can result in an arthritic condition. Temporal arteritis is felt to be very similar to (if not a characteristic condition of) polymyalgia rheumatica.

TA is an autoimmune disease; for unknown reasons, the immune system attacks connective tissue and other parts of the body. It usually affects people who had previously been in perfectly good health, so it can be emotionally overwhelming. The average age of onset is 70, and it affects twice as many women as men. Doctors use a variety of medicines to treat TA, including corticosteroids and medicines to suppress the immune system.

11

◇

A Look to the Future

Finally, after suffering through the pain, enduring the frustration of not being able to do what you want to do, feeling old before your time, and wondering just how bad it's going to get, you can *do* something about your osteoarthritis! It *is* possible to relieve and even cure your osteoarthritis with glucosamine, chondroitin sulfates, and the rest of the Arthritis Cure. And there may be even more ways to attack the problem in the future. New methods of curing joint degeneration are rapidly taking shape in laboratories and research centers around the world.

Possibilities for the Future

Arthritis researchers have made tremendous progress in the quest to replace or repair damaged cartilage. Arteparon and Rumalon are two promising new trademarked substances, both related to chondroitin sulfates. Arteparon is purified glycosaminoglycan (GAG) polysulfate taken from the tracheas and lungs of cows, while Rumalon is a GAG-peptide complex made from calf cartilage and bone marrow. Injected into either a muscle or an artery or directly into the joint, both have successfully relieved osteoarthritis pain while enhancing cartilage healing. Certain osteoarthritic changes have been reversed in some patients using these preparations, and the vast majority have had no significant side effects (other than pain from the needle used to administer the medicine). It's important to remember, however, that any joint injection can result in infection, and some people have had allergic reactions to Arteparon. (A new processing technique should reduce the incidence of allergies.) Arteparon is not yet available for use in the United States. (A related product called Adequan, also trademarked, is approved in the United States for use on animals when prescribed by veterinarians.) Additional double-blinded studies on these products and FDA approval are needed before a general recommendation for their use can be made.

Meanwhile, the art of transplanting cartilage is steadily improving. Scientists in Philadelphia have successfully transplanted bone and cartilage cells from the marrow of one mouse into another.[1] And in 1995 a police officer became one of the first American recipients of a therapy called *autologous chondrocyte implantation*, or *ACI* for short.[2] This officer had been viciously kicked in both knees and knocked to the ground when he stopped a drunk driver on a Halloween night. Significantly disabled for the next two years, he was forced to rely on prescription drugs to ease his constant pain. Total knee replacement was considered, but he felt that it was too costly and painful. Besides, it would restore only partial mobility to his knees, and would probably have to be redone in another ten years. Instead, he opted for ACI. Doctors took healthy cartilage from one part of his knee, using it to cultivate a healthy, living graft. The graft was then implanted into the damaged joint. It takes at least a year before results can be assessed so as of this writing it's still too early to declare the procedure a success, but doctors are optimistic about the outcome.

ACI originated and has been used successfully in Sweden, mostly for osteoarthritis of the knee.[3] Swedish doctors are also experimenting with its use on defects of the cartilage of the ankle and shoulder joints. Better results are obtained when the patient is younger and has small, isolated cartilage defects involving certain bones (articular cartilage on the femur seems to respond better than cartilage behind the knee).[4] As of this writing, approximately 60 Americans have undergone ACI, but since it's such a new procedure we don't know if this new cartilage lasts for more than a couple of years, or if it will break down under the pressure of everyday use. We do know, however, that this approach seems to be effective only for secondary osteoarthritis (e.g., cartilage injury due to trauma), not for primary osteoarthritis.

Taking another tact, researchers at the Massachusetts Institute of Technology (MIT) have been working with "test tube cartilage."[5] So far, they have been able to grow a stiff but flexible material that is almost identical to normal cartilage. We don't yet know if this "test tube cartilage" can be transplanted into damaged joints, and whether or not it will withstand the stress of everyday life, but the possibilities are intriguing.

Another exciting development in cartilage regeneration is the development of a cartilage-generating substance called *chondrogeneron*. Chondrogeneron is a combination of *transforming growth factor beta (TGFβ)* and fibrinogen, which "glues" the TGFβ to the damaged cartilage. Chondrogeneron has been found to promote cartilage growth and to repair cartilage defects in laboratory animals.[6] Like cartilage transplants and "test tube cartilage," this cartilage-generating substance may become an effective treatment in the future.

Several doctors in the United States have also been experimenting with *meniscus transplants*. They theorize that restoring a damaged meniscus (the cushioning cartilage in the knee) with either donated tissue or synthetic materials may help to normalize the joint forces and prevent or slow osteoarthritis. More study is needed before the medical community will accept this procedure as a standard treatment.

Possibilities for the future are nearly unlimited. We may have special "vaccines" able to bind up the "cartilage busting" enzymes and stop them in their tracks, or techniques for inserting healthy genes into damaged cartilage, replacing the defective cells that produce inferior material. Given enough time and a little bit of luck, we may conquer osteoarthritis once and for all.

An Exciting, Effective Approach We Can Use Today

Fortunately, we don't have to wait for these experimental approaches to go through years of testing and refinement before we can attack the osteoarthritis problem. With the Arthritis Cure, we already have a simple, safe, and effective means of encouraging cartilage repair. By following the simple 9-step plan, you should be able to significantly decrease, if not totally eradicate, your osteoarthritis-related pain and other symptoms, while possibly preventing onset of the disease in your other healthy joints.

It *is* possible to quell the pain and overcome the disability of osteoarthritis. The program is simple—all you have to do is get started!

Glossary

Active exercise   Exercise in which muscles are actively contracted by the patient without assistance from a therapist.

Active assisted exercise   Exercise in which muscles are actively contracted by the patient with assistance from a therapist.

Aerobic exercise   Physical activity that requires increased amounts of oxygen to be delivered to the muscles and tissues. This form of exercise helps to increase cardiovascular fitness.

Allograft   Tissue transplanted from an outside source (that is, another individual).

Analgesic   A drug such as acetaminophen that is used to relieve pain but has no effect on inflammation.

Anaphylaxis   A severe, sometimes fatal allergic reaction to the ingestion or injection of a substance.

Antioxidant   Compounds such as carotenoids, vitamin C, vitamin E, and selenium that prevent free radical damage to the body.

Antipyretic   A drug used to reduce fever, such as aspirin.

Arthroplasty   Surgical reconstruction or replacement of a joint.

Articular cartilage   The spongy, slick material that covers bone ends where they meet in a joint.

Ascorbate   A particular form of vitamin C.

Autograft   Tissue taken from one part of an individual's body and transplanted to another part.

Autologous chondrocyte implantation (ACI)   A surgical procedure whereby healthy cartilage is used to cultivate a graft, which is implanted into a damaged joint.

Bioflavonoids   A group of substances found in virtually all plant foods that is essential to the health of the capillary walls, as well as for the metabolism of vitamin C.

Biomechanics   The study of mechanical forces exerted on the body by movement.

Bouchard's nodes   Enlargement of the joints in the middle of the fingers. This is an occasional feature of osteoarthritis.

Cartilage   A gel-like, rubbery tissue capping the ends of the bones that meet in a joint. An excellent shock absorber, it is made of collagen and proteoglycans and protects the bone ends from wearing against each other.

Cartilage matrix   The "birthplace" of healthy cartilage.

Chondrocytes Cells that form the cartilage.

Chondrogeneron A combination of transforming growth factor beta (TGFβ) and fibrinogen ("glues" TGFβ to damaged cartilage), which promotes cartilage growth in laboratory animals.

Chondroitin sulfates Naturally occurring substances that inhibit the enzymes that can degrade cartilage, while helping to attract fluid to the proteoglycan molecules.

Chondroprotective Anything that can protect healthy cartilage cells from damage.

Collagen A vital structural protein found in cartilage that provides a dense "netting" to contain the proteoglycans, which attract and hold water in the tissue. It also provides the cartilage with elasticity and shock-absorbing properties. Cartilage is the supporting structure for the body's cells.

Corticosteroid An agent used to prevent or reduce inflammation that can have dangerous side effects such as hypertension, osteoporosis, immune system damage, and many others.

Crepitus Crackling or crunching sounds made by the bones in the joints upon movement.

Depression Feelings of sadness, despair, or discouragement that can range from mild to severe and occur on a chronic, recurrent basis or as a one-time event. Differs from "the blues."

* * *

Eburnation   Abnormal bone denseness often seen in osteoarthritis.

Fat-soluble vitamins   Vitamins that only dissolve in fat tissues and stay in the body much longer than water-soluble vitamins. Vitamins A, D, E, and K are fat-soluble.

Fatty acid   An organic acid that is either manufactured by the body or must be supplied by the diet. Examples of fatty acids include linoleic, linolenic, and arachidonic acid.

Free radical   An unstable molecule created by normal metabolic processes or by exposure to cigarette smoke, radiation, or other environmental factors. These molecules damage healthy tissues by "stealing" electrons from other molecules, thereby undermining them.

Gastrointestinal   Of or pertaining to the organs of the digestive tract, from mouth to anus.

Glucosamine   The key substance that determines how many proteoglycan (water-holding) molecules are formed in the cartilage. The greater the amount of glucosamine, the greater the amount of proteoglycans.

Glycosaminoglycans (GAGs)   Important proteins in cartilage that bind the water in the cartilage matrix.

Graft   Tissue or an organ transplanted from one site to another on the same individual.

* * *

Half-life The length of time a drug stays in the body until half of the initial concentration has been metabolized or eliminated.

Heberden's nodes Disfigurement of the joints of the hand nearest to the fingertips. Common in long-standing osteoarthritis.

Inflammation Response of the body's tissues to irritation or injury, often characterized by pain, swelling, redness, and heat.

Isometric exercise Exercise in which muscle tension is increased by applying pressure against stable resistance (for example, pressing your hands together). The joints are not moved. (This is a commonly prescribed type of exercise for arthritis patients.)

Isotonic exercise Exercise (e.g., weight lifting) in which muscle is contracted and joint is moved. Best suited for people without inflamed joints.

Manganese Mineral that increases the effectiveness of both glucosamine and chondroitin sulfates and is important in synthesis of cartilage.

Mineral An inorganic substance such as manganese or zinc that is needed in small amounts for proper growth and functioning of the body.

Monoamine-oxidase (MAO) inhibitors A class of antidepressants that protect "mood-elevating" substances (such as norepinephrine) from breaking down, thus increasing their levels in the body.

*   *   *

Neurotransmitter Chemical "switches" in the nervous system that carry messages from one nerve cell to the next.

NSAIDs Nonsteroidal anti-inflammatory drugs commonly used to alleviate the pain and inflammation associated with osteoarthritis.

Osteoblast Cells that produce bone tissue.

Osteoclast Cells that break down and aid in the resorption of bone tissue.

Osteophytes Bone spurs. Usually form at the margin of osteoarthritic joints.

Osteotomy Surgical removal of part of the subchondral bone to realign the bone position.

Passive exercise Movement in which the muscles are moved by an outside source, such as a therapist or equipment.

Pharmaceutical grade The level of purity that is consistent with FDA-approved laboratory standards.

Prednisone An artificial cortisone drug used to treat rheumatoid arthritis, allergic reactions, and inflammation.

Prostaglandin A group of hormonelike fatty acids that are produced in the body in small amounts and are responsible for the inflammation process, among many other functions.

Proteoglycans Large water-binding molecules, consisting of proteins and sugars, that act as major building blocks of cartilage.

*   *   *

Range-of-motion exercises Exercises designed to reduce stiffness and increase the flexibility of the joints. (The "range of motion" is the extent to which an individual's joints normally move.)

Resistive exercise Actively contracting a muscle while working against mechanical or manual pressure.

Selective serotonin reuptake inhibitors (SSRIs) A type of antidepressant that selectively affects the part of the brain influenced by serotonin, thereby lifting depression with fewer side effects than earlier antidepressants.

Stress Any physical, emotional, economic, social, or other factor that requires a bodily response or change. Continual stress brings about widespread changes in body function and often has an adverse effect on the health.

Subchondral bone The bone located directly under joint cartilage.

Subchondral cysts Fluid-filled pockets in the bone with osteoarthritis.

Synovial fluid A lubricating fluid found inside the joint which allows for smooth joint motion.

Synovial membrane (also called synovium) The lining of moveable joints that secretes synovial fluid.

Tricyclic antidepressants The earliest form of antidepressant developed, these drugs manipulate norepinephrine (a "mood elevator" in the brain) and can be either sedating or stimulating.

Vitamins   Any group of organic compounds that the body needs for normal growth, development, and metabolism. Most cannot be synthesized by the body so must be supplied by the diet. The lack of a vitamin can cause a deficiency disease.

Water-soluble vitamins   Vitamins that easily dissolve in water, and therefore can be eliminated from the body in a short time. Water-soluble vitamins include the B vitamins and vitamin C.

References

◇

Chapter 1: Can Osteoarthritis Be Cured?

1. Lewis, R. "Arthritis: Modern Treatment for That Old Pain in the Joints." *FDA Consumer* 25:18–26, July/August 1991.

2. McKenzie, L. S., Horsburgh, B. A., Ghosh, P., and Taylor, T. K. F. "Osteoarthrosis: Uncertain Rationale for Anti-inflammatory Drug Therapy." *Lancet* 1:908–909, 1976.

3. Vidal y Plana, R. R., Bizzardi, D., and Rovati, A. L. "Articular Cartilage Pharmacology: In Vitro Studies on Glucosamine and Non-steroidal Anti-inflammatory Drugs." *Pharmacological Research Communications* 10(6):557–569, 1978.

4. Palmoski, J. J., and Brandt, K. D. "Effects of Some Non-steroidal Anti-inflammatory Drugs on Proteoglycan Metabolism and Organization in Canine Articular Cartilage." *Arthritis and Rheumatism* 23: 1010–1020, 1980.

5. Moskowitz, R. *Osteoarthritis Diagnosis and Management*, Introduction. Philadelphia: W. B. Saunders Company, 1992, pp. 1–6.

6. Ibid. Chapter 8: Osteoarthritis Symptoms and Signs, pp. 149–154.

7. Mankin, H. J. *Arthritis Surgery*, Chapter 25: Clinical Features of Osteoarthritis. Philadelphia: W. B. Saunders Company, 1994, pp. 469–479.

8. Liang, M. H. "A Joint Endeavor." *Harvard Health Letter* 17(6):1–4, April 1992.

9. "Joints Feel the Weight." *Prevention* 41:10, February 1989.

10. Felson, D. T., et al. "Obesity and Knee Osteoarthritis: The Framingham Study." *Annals of Internal Medicine* 109:18–24, July 1, 1988.

11. Weiss, R. "Geneticists to Arthritics: A Gene's the Rub." *Science News* 138:148, 1990.

12. Griffin, M., et al. "Practical Management of Osteoarthritis." *Archives of Family Medicine* 4:1049–1055, December 1995.

13. Mankin. Op cit. Chapter 25: "Clinical Features of Osteoarthritis," pp. 469–479.

14. Swedberg, J. A., and Steinbauer, J. R. "Osteoarthritis." *American Family Physician* 45(2):557–568, February 1992.

15. Peyron, J. C. *Osteoarthritis Diagnosis and Management*, Chapter 1: The Epidemiology of Osteoarthritis. Philadelphia: W. B. Saunders Company, 1992, pp. 9–27.

16. Tsang, J. K. "Update on Osteoarthritis." *Canadian Family Physician* 36(614):539–544, 1990.

17. *Arthritis Information: Rheumatoid Arthritis.* Atlanta, Ga.: The Arthritis Foundation, Brochure No. 4020, March 1995.

18. *Arthritis Information: Osteoarthritis.* Atlanta, Ga.: The Arthritis Foundation, Brochure No. 4040, May 1995.

19. Mankin. Op. cit. Chapter 25: Clinical Features of Osteoarthritis, pp. 469–479.

20. Swedberg and Steinbauer. Op. cit.

21. Bland. Op. cit.

22. Liang, M. H., and Fortin, P. "Management of Osteoarthritis of the Hip and Knee." *The Journal of the American Medical Association* 325(2):125–127, July 11, 1991.

23. Bland. Op cit.

24. Adams, M. E. "Cartilage Research and Treatment of Osteoarthritis." *Current Opinions in Rheumatology* 4:552–559, 1992.

Chapter 2: When Joints Go Bad

1. Brandt, K. D., and Mankin, H. J. *Arthritis Surgery*, Chapter 24: Pathogenesis of Osteoarthritis. Philadelphia: W. B. Saunders Company, 1994, pp. 450–468.

2. Buckwalter, J. A., et al. "Restoration of Injured or Degenerated Articular Cartilage." *Journal of the American Academy of Orthopaedic Surgeons* 2(4):192–201, July/August 1994.

3. Caplan, A. I. "Cartilage." *Scientific American* 251(1):84–97, October 1984.

4. Sledge, C. B. *Arthritis Surgery*, Chapter 1: Biology of the Joint. Philadelphia: W. B. Saunders Company, 1994, pp. 1–21.

5. Kushner, L. (The Arthritis Foundation). *Understanding Arthritis: What It Is, How to Treat It, How to Cope With It*. New York: Macmillan General Reference, 1984, pp. 60–61.

6. Buckwalter et al. Op. cit.

7. Meachin, G., and Brooke G. *Osteoarthritis Diagnosis and Management*, Chapter 2: The Pathology of Osteoarthritis. Philadelphia: W. B. Saunders Company, 1992, pp. 29–42.

8. *Arthritis Information: Osteonecrosis*. Atlanta, Ga.: The Arthritis Foundation, Brochure No. 9337, May 1994.

Chapter 3: New Hope for Beating Osteoarthritis

1. Müeller-Faßbender, H., et al. "Glucosamine Sulfate Compared to Ibuprofen in Osteoarthritis of the Knee." *Osteoarthritis and Cartilage* 2:61–69, 1994.

2. Crolle, G., and D'Este, E. "Glucosamine Sulphate for the Management of Arthrosis: A Controlled Clinical Investigation." *Current Medical Research and Opinion* 7(2):104–109, 1980.

3. Dovanti, A., Bignamini, A. A., and Rovati, A. L. "Therapeutic Activity of Oral Glucosamine Sulphate in Osteoarthrosis: A Placebo-Controlled Double-Blind Investigation." *Clinical Therapeutics* 3(4):266–272, 1980.

4. Pujalte, J. M., Llavore, E. P., and Ylescupidez, F. R. "Double-blind Clinical Evaluation of Oral Glucosamine Sulphate in the Basic Treatment of Osteoarthrosis." *Current Medical Research and Opinion* 7(2): 110–114, 1980.

5. Dovanti et al. Op. Cit.

6. Pujalte et al. Op. cit.

7. Vajaradul, Y. "Double-blind Clinical Evaluation of Intra-articular Glucosamine in Outpatients with Gonarthrosis." *Clinical Therapeutics* 3(5):260+, 1980.

8. Crolle, G., and D'Este, E. "Glucosamine Sulphate for the Management of Arthrosis: A Controlled Clinical Investigation." *Current Medical Research and Opinion* 7(2):104–109, 1980.

9. Tapadinhas, M. J., Rivera, I. C., and Bignamini, A. A. "Oral Glucosamine Sulphate in the Management of Arthrosis: Report on a Multi-centre Open Investigation in Portugal." *Pharmatherapeutica* 3(3):157–168, 1982.

10. Vaz, A. L. "Double-blind Clinical Evaluation of the Relative Efficacy of Ibuprofen and Glucosamine Sulphate in the Management of Osteoarthrosis of the Knee in Out-patients." *Current Medical Research and Opinion* 8(3):145–149, 1982.

11. Faßbender, H. M., et al. "Glucosamine Sulfate Compared to Ibuprofen in Osteoarthritis of the Knee." *Osteoarthritis and Cartilage* 2(1):61–69, 1994.

12. D'Ambrosio, E., et al. "Glucosamine Sulfate: A

Controlled Clinical Investigation in Arthrosis." *Pharmatherapeutica* 2(8):504+, 1981.

13. Caplan, A. I. "Cartilage." *Scientific American* 251(1):84–97, October 1984.

14. Soldani, G., and Romagnoli, J. "Experimental and Clinical Pharmacology of Glycosaminoglycans (GAGs)." *Drugs in Experimental and Clinical Research* 18(1):81–85, 1991.

15. Rovetta, G. "Galactosaminoglycuronoglycan Sulfate (Matrix) in Therapy of Tibiofibular Osteoarthritis of the Knee." *Drugs in Experimental and Clinical Research* 18(1):53–57, 1991.

16. Soldani and Romagnoli. Op. cit.

17. Prudden, J. F., and Balassa, L. L. "The Biological Activity of Bovine Cartilage Preparations." *Seminars on Arthritis and Rheumatism* 3(4):287+, 1974.

18. Rovetta. Op. cit.

19. Pipitone, V. R. "Chondroprotection with Chondroitin Sulfate." *Drugs in Experimental and Clinical Research* 17(1):3–7, 1991.

20. Oliviero, U., et al. "Effects of the Treatment with Matrix on Elderly People with Chronic Articular Degeneration." *Drugs in Experimental and Clinical Research* 17(1):45–51, 1991.

21. Mazières, B., et al. "Le Chondroitin Sulfate Dayns le Traitement de la Gonarthrose et de la Coxarthrose." *Rev. Rheum. Mal Ostéoartic* 59(7–8):466–472, 1992.

22. Kerzberg, E. M., et al. "Combination of Glycosaminoglycans and Acetylsalicylic Acid in Knee Osteoarthrosis." *Scandinavian Journal of Rheumatology* 16:377–380, 1987.

23. Dixon, J., et al. *Second-Line Agents in the Treatment of Rheumatic Diseases.* New York: Marcel Dekker, 1992, pp. 363–427.

Chapter 4: The Arthritis Cure

1. Bucci, L. R. *Nutrition Applied to Injury Rehabilitation and Sports Medicine.* Boca Raton, Fla.: CRC Press, 1994, pp. 140–149.

2. Ibid., pp. 95–102.

3. Fries, J. F., et al. "Running and the Development of Disability with Age." *Annals of Internal Medicine* 121:502–509, 1994.

4. Bunning, R. D., and Materson, R. S. "A Rational Program of Exercise for Patients with Osteoarthritis." *Seminars in Arthritis and Rheumatism* 21(3):33–43, December 1991.

5. Bucci. Op. cit., pp. 95–102.

6. Murray, M. T. *Arthritis: How You Can Benefit from Diet, Vitamins, Minerals, Herbs, Exercise and Other Natural Methods.* Rocklin, Calif.: Prima Publishing, 1994, pp. 66–73.

7. Felson, D. T., et al. "Weight Loss Reduces the Risk for Symptomatic Knee Osteoarthritis in Women: The Framingham Study." *Annals of Internal Medicine* 116:535–539, 1992.

8. Traut, E. F., and Thrift, C. B. "Obesity in Arthritis: Related Factors, Dietary Factors." *Journal of the American Geriatric Society* 17:710–717, 1969.

9. Fox, S., and Fox, B. *Beyond Positive Thinking.* Carson, Calif.: Hay House, 1991, p. 64.

Chapter 5: The Problem with Painkillers

1. Gay, G. "Another Side Effect of NSAIDs." *Journal of the American Medical Association* 264(20):2677–2678, November 28, 1990.

2. Sandler, D. P. "Analgesic Use and Chronic Renal Disease." *The New England Journal of Medicine* 320:1238–1243, 1989.

3. Garnett, L. R. "Strong Medicine." *Harvard Health Letter*, April 1995, pp. 4–6.

4. Calabro, J. J. *Osteoarthritis Diagnosis and Man-*

agement, Chapter 18: Principles of Drug Therapy. Philadelphia: W. B. Saunders Company, 1992, pp. 317–322.

5. Garnett. Op. cit.

6. Brooks, P. M., and Day, R. O. "Nonsteroidal Anti-inflammatory Drugs—Differences and Similarities." *The New England Journal of Medicine* 324(24): 1716–1725, June 13, 1991.

7. Novak, K. K., et al. *Drug Facts and Comparisons.* St. Louis, Mo.: Facts and Comparisons, Inc., 1995.

8. Hendler, N., and Kolodny, A. L. "Using Medication Wisely in Chronic Pain." *Patient Care*, 26:125–139, May 15, 1992.

9. Hodgkinson, R., and Woolf, D. "A Five-Year Clinical Trial of Indomethacin in Osteoarthritis of the Hip Joint." ACTA Orhtop Scand. 50:169, 1979.

10. Bradley, J. D., et al. "Comparison of an Anti-inflammatory Dose of Ibuprofen, an Analgesic Dose of Ibuprofen, and Acetaminophen in the Treatment of Patients with Osteoarthritis of the Knee." *The New England Journal of Medicine* 325:87–91, 1991.

11. Hench, P. K., and Willkens, R. F. "Choosing the Right NSAID for Joint Pain." *Patient Care*, 28(76):76–108, 1994.

12. Calabro. Op. cit.

13. Brooks and Day. Op. cit.

14. Ibid.

15. Calabro. Op. cit.

16. Stehlin, D. "How to Take Your Medicine—Nonsteroidal Anti-inflammatory Drugs." *FDA Consumer* pp. 33–34, June 1990.

Chapter 6: Exercise That *Helps*, Not Hurts

1. Gecht, M. R., et al. "A Survey of Exercise Beliefs and Exercise Habits Among People with Arthritis."

Arthritis Care and Research, 9(2):82–88, April 1996.

2. Rock, M. "A Strong Case for Strength Training." *Arthritis Today* 8(6):45–50, November/December 1994.

3. Bunning, R. D., and Materson, R. S. Op. cit.

4. Rock. Op. cit.

5. Morrow, S. "Take It in Stride: Walking Is Fun for Fall." *Arthritis Today* 8(5):59–61, September/October 1994.

6. *Arthritis Information: Exercise and Your Arthritis.* Atlanta, Ga.: The Arthritis Foundation, Brochure No. 835–5455, January 1996.

7. McNeal, R. L. "Aquatic Therapy for Patients with Rheumatic Disease." *Rheumatic Disease Clinics of North America* 16(4):915–943, November 1990.

8. Centerpiece. "Stretching, the Truth." *UC Berkeley Wellness Letter* 11:4–6, November 1994.

Chapter 7: Healthy Eating Really Counts

1. Bucci. Op. cit., pp. 69–76.

2. Nierenberg, C. "The Antioxidant Avalanche." *Arthritis Today*, January/February 1996, pp. 48–50.

3. Adderly, B. A. *The Complete Guide to Pills.* New York: Ballantine Books, 1996, p. 1061.

4. Ibid., p. 1066.

5. Ibid., p. 1067.

6. Fox, S., and Fox, B. *Immune for Life.* Rocklin, Calif.: Prima Publishing, p. 256.

7. Travers, R. L., and Rennie, G. C. "Clinical Trial—Boron and Arthritis. The Results of a Double-blind Pilot Study." *Townsend Letter for Doctors*, June 1990, pp. 360–366.

8. Bucci. Op. cit., pp. 205–208.

9. Ibid.

10. Williams, S. R. *Nutrition and Diet Therapy.* St. Louis, Mo.: Times Mirror/Mosby, 1985, pp. 516–518.

11. Dunkin, M. A. "Medicines vs. Nutrients." *Ar-*

thritis Today, January/February 1991, pp. 46–47.

12. Ibid.

13. Ibid.

14. Ibid.

15. Murray, M. *Arthritis: How You Can Benefit from Diet, Vitamins, Minerals, Herbs, Exercise and Other Natural Methods*. Rocklin, Calif.: Prima Publishing, 1994, pp. 66–72.

16. Ibid.

17. Olivenstein, L. "Craving Cure." *Arthritis Today* 10(3)33–39, May/June 1996.

Chapter 8: Beating the Blues

1. O'Koon, M. "Out of the Dark." *Arthritis Today* 9(1)34–40, January/February 1996.

2. Ibid.

3. Ibid.

4. Fries, J. F. *Arthritis: A Take Care of Yourself Health Guide*. Reading, Mass.: Addison Wesley, 1995, pp. 238–239.

5. O'Koon. Op. cit.

6. Brandt, K. D. *Arthritis Surgery*, Chapter 26: Management of Osteoarthritis. Philadelphia: W. B. Saunders Company, 1994, pp. 480–494.

7. Mondimore, F. M. *Depression: The Mood Disease*. Baltimore, Md.: The Johns Hopkins University Press, 1993.

8. Dexter, P., and Brandt, K. "Distribution and Predictors of Depressive Symptoms of Osteoarthritis." *The Journal of Rheumatology* 21(2):279–286, 1994.

9. Orlock, C. "The Healing Power of Touch." *Arthritis Today* 8(6):34–37, November/December 1994.

Chapter 9: You *Can* Prevent Osteoarthritis

1. Rocklin. Op. cit.

2. Bucci. Op. cit., pp. 69–76.

3. Ibid., pp. 205–208.

4. Dunkin. Op. cit.

5. Felson, D., et al. "Weight Loss Reduces Risk for Symptomatic Knee Osteoarthritis in Women." *Annals of Internal Medicine* 116(7):535–539, April 1, 1992.

6. Delaney, L. "Stop Arthritis Now!" *Prevention,* January 1994, pp. 60–67, 126.

7. Theodosakis, J., and Davis, R. "Prevention and Treatment of Athletic Injuries." *Exercise and Fitness* (Canyon Ranch Publication), 1993, pp. 1–8.

8. Felson. Op. cit.

9. Felson, D. T., et al. "Obesity and Knee Osteoarthritis. The Framingham Study." *Annals of Internal Medicine* 109:18–24, July 1988.

Chapter 10: The Arthritis Primer

1. *Arthritis Information: Ankylosing Spondylitis.* Atlanta, Ga.: The Arthritis Foundation, Brochure No. 9050, October 1995.

2. *Understanding Arthritis.* Op. cit., pp. 161–175.

3. Fries. Op. cit., pp. 42–47.

4. *Understanding Arthritis.* Op. cit., pp. 236–247.

5. Fries. Op. cit., pp. 91–93.

6. Vierck, E. H. *Keys to Understanding Arthritis.* Hauppauge, N.Y.: Barron's Educational Series, 1991, pp. 57–58.

7. *Arthritis Information: Gout.* Atlanta, Ga.: The Arthritis Foundation, Brochure No. 835–5235, February 1996.

8. *Understanding Arthritis.* Op. cit., pp. 195–203.

9. Fries. Op. cit., pp. 53–58.

10. *Understanding Arthritis.* Op. cit., pp. 210–216.

11. Vierck. Op. cit., pp. 33–35.

12. *Understanding Arthritis.* Op. cit., pp. 182–194.

13. Fries. Op. cit., pp. 27–32.

14. *Understanding Arthritis.* Op. cit., pp. 204–209.

15. Fries. Op. cit., pp. 59–61.

16. *Arthritis Information: Psoriatic Arthritis.* Atlanta, Ga.: The Arthritis Foundation, Brochure No. 9053, October 1995.

17. *Understanding Arthritis.* Op. cit., pp. 217–222.

18. Fries. Op. cit., pp. 37–40.

19. *Arthritis Information: Reiter's Syndrome.* Atlanta, Ga.: The Arthritis Foundation, Brochure No. 4350, June 1994.

20. *Understanding Arthritis.* Op. cit., pp. 176–181.

21. Fries. Op. cit., pp. 47–51.

22. *Arthritis Information: Rheumatoid Arthritis.* Op. cit.

23. *Understanding Arthritis.* Op. cit., pp. 126–133.

24. Fries. Op. cit., pp. 19–26.

25. Vierck. Op. cit., pp. 17–21.

26. *Understanding Arthritis.* Op. cit., p. 229.

27. Fries. Op. cit., pp. 102–104.

28. Vierck. Op. cit., pp. 39–41.

29. *Arthritis Information: Paget's Disease.* Atlanta, Ga.: The Arthritis Foundation, Brochure No. 9064, November 1992.

30. Vierck. Op. cit., pp. 50–52.

31. *Arthritis Information: Polymyalgia Rheumatica.* Atlanta, Ga.: The Arthritis Foundation, Brochure No. 4330, September 1995.

32. *Understanding Arthritis.* Op. cit., pp. 223–227.

33. Fries. Op. cit., pp. 83–86.

34. *Arthritis Information: Myositis.* Atlanta, Ga.: The Arthritis Foundation, Brochure No. 4390, September 1995.

35. *Understanding Arthritis.* Op. cit., pp. 154–160.

36. Fries. Op. cit., pp. 86–90.

37. *Arthritis Information: Scleroderma.* Atlanta, Ga.: The Arthritis Foundation, Brochure No. 9051, September 1995.

38. *Understanding Arthritis*. Op. cit., pp. 143–153.

39. Vierck. Op. cit., pp. 42–44.

40. *Arthritis Information: Sjögren's Syndrome*. Atlanta, Ga.: The Arthritis Foundation, Brochure No. 9328, August 1995.

41. *Understanding Arthritis*. Op. cit., p. 27.

42. *Arthritis Information: Lupus*. Atlanta, Ga.: The Arthritis Foundation, Brochure No. 9052, September 1995.

43. *Understanding Arthritis*. Op. cit., pp. 134–142.

44. Fries. Op. cit., pp. 32–36.

45. Vierck. Op. cit., pp. 23–26.

46. *Understanding Arthritis*. Op. cit., pp. 226–227.

Chapter 11: A Look to the Future

1. The Arthritis Foundation. "New Method to Replace Cartilage/Bone." Public Information Memo, December 12, 1995, pp. 1–2.

2. Kalb, C., and Cowley, G. "Hope for Damaged Joints." *Newsweek*, January 29, 1996, p. 55.

3. Brittberg, M., et al. "Treatment of Deep Cartilage Defects in the Knee with Autologous Chondrocyte Transplantation." *The New England Journal of Medicine* 331(14):889–895, October 6, 1994.

4. "Growing a New Knee: Transplanting Cartilage." *Penn State Sports Medicine Newsletter* 3(10):1–2, June 1995.

5. Skerrett, P. J. "Growing New Cartilage to Fight Arthritis." *Technology Review* 96:10–12, April 1993.

6. The Arthritis Foundation. "Cartilage Growth Factor (TGFB) in Osteoarthritis." Public Information Memo, February 24, 1994.

Index

If you would like to contact Dr. Theodosakis, please write him at:

Publicity Department
c/o Dr. Jason Theodosakis
St.Martin's Press
175 Fifth Avenue
New York, NY 10010

About the Authors

DR. JASON THEODOSAKIS
Dr. Jason Theodosakis (or Dr. Theo, as he is known) is an Assistant Clinical Professor at the University of Arizona College of Medicine in Tucson, Arizona.

He is board-certified in preventive medicine and public health and fellowship-trained in sports medicine. Dr. Theo received his medical degree from the University of Health Sciences/Chicago Medical School. In addition, he graduated summa cum laude with master's degrees in both Public Health and Exercise Physiology from the University of Arizona.

BRENDA ADDERLY, M.H.A.
Brenda Adderly, M.H.A., is a health-care researcher, writer, and consultant who has worked in the federal, not-for-profit, and for-profit sectors of health care. Her assignments have included: staff assistant under Dr. C. Everett Koop; HMO and physician group marketing; and co-founding a managed-care consulting firm. She is the author of

The Complete Guide to Pills, a consumer guide that profiles the most commonly prescribed drugs.

Brenda holds a master's degree in Health Services Administration from the George Washington University in Washington, D.C.

BARRY FOX, PH.D.

Barry Fox, Ph.D., is the author of *Foods to Heal By* and *To Your Health,* and the best-selling coauthor of many other books, including *The Beverly Hills Medical Diet, Alternative Healing,* and *The Healthy Prostate.* A noted inspirational and health speaker who appears in person and on radio and television, Barry has traveled around the country teaching people how to live young and stay healthy to a very old age.